A history of the **University of Bristol Dental School** and its site

Chris Stephens

University of Bristol Dental Alumni Association

www.bristoldentalalumni.co.uk

First published in 2012 by C.D.Stephens
for the University of Bristol Dental Alumni Association
c/o Clinical Dean's Office
Dental School
Lower Maudlin Street
Bristol
BS1 2LY

ISBN 978-0-9549861-5-5

Cover design by J.D.Stephens

Typeset in Myriad Pro 11/15
by Georgina Pensri, West Sussex, England

Printed and bound in the United Kingdom
by Euro-Print Limited, Cardiff, Wales

Contents

List of Figures

To my wife

Published to mark the centenary of the first Bristol dental undergraduate to qualify BDS UBrist.

Acknowledgements

The author has depended heavily on earlier accounts of the School notably the two accounts by Bishop Saunders published by the Bristol Royal Infirmary in 1964 and 1965 and that of Dr. Hugh Levers of 1989 which is retained by the University. I have also benefited from the excellent records held in the Special Collections of the University of Bristol and I am indebted to Michael Richardson, Senior Assistant Librarian, Special Collections, for help in accessing these. Others to be thanked include Gail Boyle of the City Museum Bristol, Jane Southway of the Bristol charity Above and Beyond, Ms Patricia Burke LDS U Brist. and Mr Michael Platt BDS U Brist.

I am particularly grateful to my former colleagues: Chris Stephenson for his many photographs of the dental school site, Professor David Berry for the photograph of the Dental Laboratory in the 1930s, and Iain Hathorn and Professor Alan Harrison for proof reading. Gordon Gray, the current Dental Dean, has been very helpful in answering my many points of details. It was Professor Robin Matthews whose talk on the history of the dental school site given at a final year dinner in 1976 inspired me to continue his work which now forms Chapter 1.

To those former students whose comments and anecdotes enliven the text my thanks. In this connection special thanks must go to the late Hugh Leech whose vivid account drawn from his diary as a dental student in the war years forms a significant part of Chapter 5.

The University of Bristol Dental Alumni Association is grateful for the support of the Dental Defence Union in the production of this book, which has been produced to mark the centenary of the Bristol BDS degree.

THE DDU

Preface

No history can ever be complete, and this account is no exception. Readers must excuse the many omissions particularly names of recent staff which have been omitted. It had been intended to include these as a list in an appendix but finding that there had been 770 academic, research and honorary staff appointed between the years 1988 and 2010 this was felt to be impracticable! I am also aware that very little has been mentioned about the evolution of technical and nursing service which I must leave to others to record.

One of the problems I found was to put what have been local issues for the Dental Hospital and School within the context of national changes within the profession, the National Health Service and University Higher Education. While perhaps not of the greatest interest to students at the time, my aim has been to explain to our graduates some of the pressures their teachers were wrestling with while at the same time dealing with the more obvious tasks of producing competent and caring clinicians. Such pressures of course applied to all dental schools but bore down more heavily on Bristol because of its very low number of University staff.

At the time of writing there is much public debate about the proposal for yet another reorganisation of the UK National Health Service. I can only observe that most of the 10 reorganisations we were subject to in my time at Bristol proved to be only half thought out . Each required a considerable period of negotiation and adjustment to overcome many unforeseen consequences in order to be of any real benefit. It is sad to reflect that while evolution has worked well for life on this planet for 400 million years, Ministers always think they have hit upon a revolutionary change which will immediately improve matters but seldom do. The changes to which Dental Schools have become subject in the recent past were invariably intended for medicine and only later did our political masters realise that they also affected dental hospitals and academic dentistry in unintended ways.

What does improve the performance of complex organisations such as a dental school, which has to meet the competing demands of teaching, service provision and research, are all the small incremental changes which are adopted by common consent. These require the continuous commitment and amicable debate among colleagues, be they staff or students. This has been the strength of the Bristol Dental School during my time.

All the proceeds from this book go to the Bristol Dental Alumni Association in its support of continuing excellence of dental education at Bristol.

Chris Stephens, Professor Emeritus in Child Dental Health, November 2011.

Chapter 1

THE BRISTOL DENTAL SCHOOL SITE

A great deal is known about the present Bristol Dental School site which originally lay on a flat area overlooking the River Frome as it flowed through a marshy valley on its way to join the River Avon to the southwest of the city. Excavations in 1973 produced flint and chert (cryptocrystalline or microfibrous sedimentary rock) artefacts from the Mesolithic, Neolithic and early Bronze Ages but probably represented episodic visits by prehistoric peoples taking advantage of low cliff terrain overlooking the flood plains of two rivers[1]. Coins and pottery recovered during these investigations also revealed that this had been one of the earliest sites of Romano-British occupation to be discovered in Bristol. This corner of the excavation could not be fully investigated as it extended beneath the roadway of Upper Maudlin Street but was dated to the 2nd – 4th centuries AD[2].

These excavations had been undertaken when the Upper Maudlin Street site became scheduled for redevelopment and was intended to investigate the mediaeval buildings of the religious foundation of Greyfriars (Friars Minor / Franciscans) which was known to exist there from earlier accounts[3].

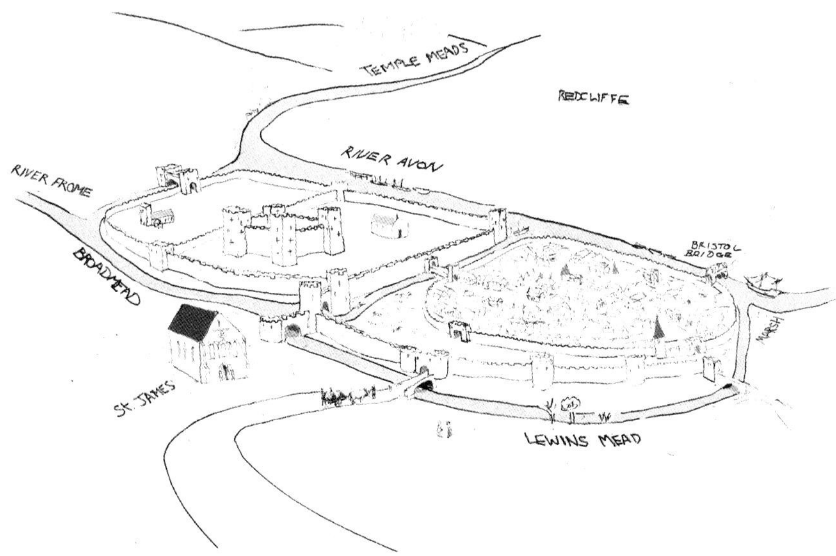

Figure 1 View from Kingsdown looking towards the city as it might have been in 1240

The order of Greyfriars first came to Bristol in about 1230 AD and took their name from the plain undyed woollen robes they wore. Around 1250 a site for the order was found below the present dental school, beside Lewin's Mead, possibly on land given by the Benedictine Prior of St. James which had been built by Robert Earl of Gloucester in 1138. (Lewin's Mead takes it name from the chamberlain of Robert 2nd Earl of Gloucester). Both these religious establishments stood outside the city which at that time was walled and protected to the south by a marshy area at the junction of the rivers Avon and Frome. It would appear that the availability of this land was due to the re-alignment of the River Frome (1240-1247). Archaeological investigations in 1973 showed that building of the Friary had been in two phases and that the first had been preceded by using material from the digging of the new channel for the Frome (St.Augustine's Trench) to raise the marshy site in order to provide solid foundations.

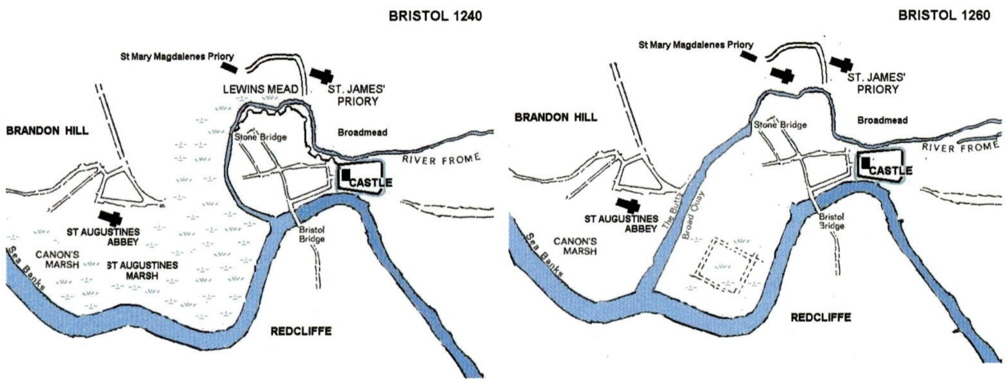

Figure 2. The course of the River Frome (a) before and (b) after the digging of St Augustines Trench.

The Greyfriars precinct was described by William Worcestre writing in 1478 as lying on the north side of Lewins Mead with "walls and gardens extending up the hill". It would appear that the site was bounded by Priors Lane (what is now Lower Maudlin Street) on the east, Upper Maudlin St on the north, Bartholomew Lane now Johnny Ball Lane on the west and Lewins Mead to the south. The friary was rebuilt extensively at the end of the 14th century. William's measurements of 1478 and 1480 describe a church of 52 metres in length with a tower 4 metres square. There was a Chapter House of 14 metres by 8 metres in 1480, (later extended to 22 metres x 8 metres) a cloister of 17 metres by 25 metres as well as the usual monastic dorter, frater, kitchens etc. These were confirmed by the excavations in 1973. The overall outline of the site based on the descriptions of William Worcestre has been suggested by Weare, (Figure 3).

Like all other religious houses the friary continued up until the dissolution of the monasteries in 1538. Weare 1893 gives a full description of the process as well as the Friary's contents at this time. The small priory of St Mary Magdalene from which

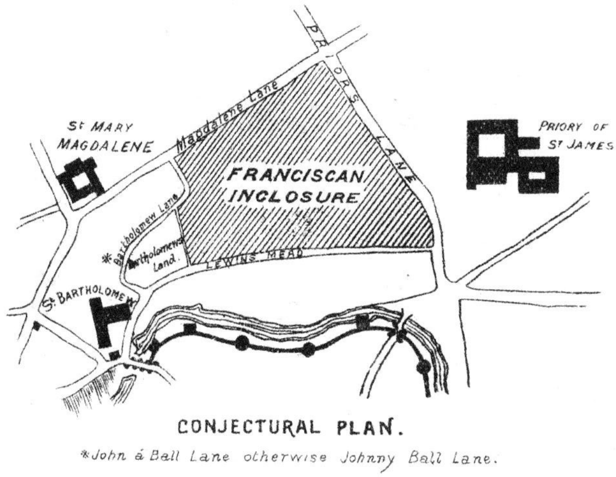

Figure 3. The plan of Greyfriars given by Weare 1893.

Maudlin Lane gets it name and which was sited at the bottom of St Michael's Hill was also surrendered at this time[4] (Figure 3).

A feature of all such monastic establishments was the construction of reliable water supplies for themselves and for the public. Several of those in Bristol have lasted into modern times[5]. The most well known is the outlet of the St. John Conduit built in 1376

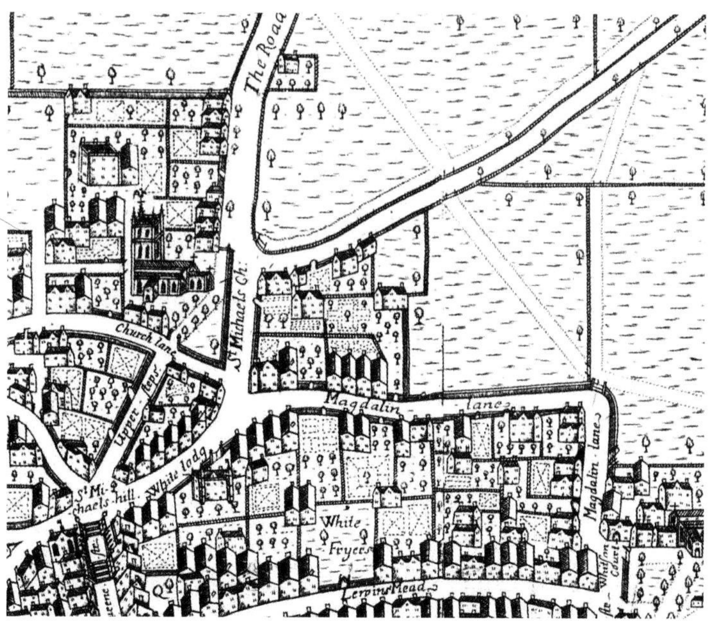

Figure 4. A section of William Millerd's map of 1673 showing Lewin's Mead and Magdalin Lane which would later become Upper and Lower Maudlin Street. The open area would later become the site of Bristol Royal Infirmary.

as an extension of a preexisting conduit This still brings water from the top of Park Street to its outlet on the north wall of the church of St. John on the Wall, Nelson Street. The Greyfriar's supply ran in a conduit from Bedford Place, Kingsdown below the site of the present Queens Building of the Royal Infirmary), to their precinct. According to Weare there was a reservoir under the houses on the north side of Upper Maudlin Street. At one time there was public access to this subterranean water channel via steps on either side of the road[6]. Following the dissolution, the Greyfriar's estate was sold to then Mayor and Corporation. The water supply was taken over by All Saints Parish. Part of this conduit, now known as All Saints Pipe was relaid in the 18th and 19th centuries below the later Moravian Chapel in Upper Maudlin Street. When the site was redeveloped in 1995 the stone which marked its course was placed in the wall of the Chapter House (Figures 5,6).

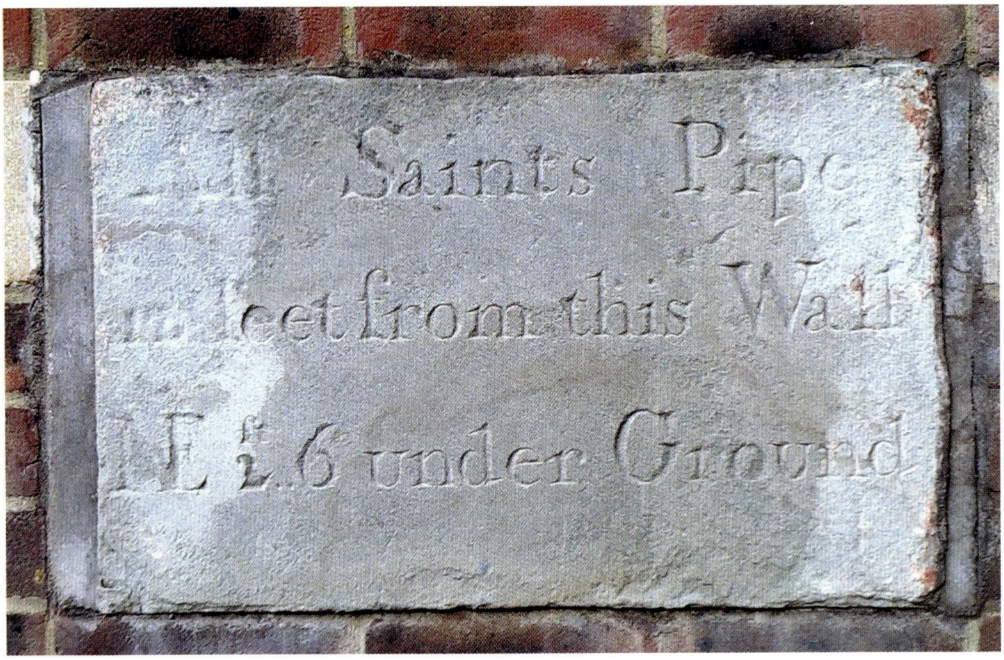

Figure 5. All Saints pipe - the stone marking the course of the former Greyfriar's conduit now reset in the wall of the Chapter House.

Knowledge of the subsequent use of the Greyfriars site is incomplete. It is known that clay pipes were manufactured in the area in the 17th and 18th centuries and it seems there was also warehousing and light industry. Two bowls this period, with blank cartouches, were recovered during excavations on the Upper Maudlin Street site in 1973.

At the end of the 19th century there were still significant remains of the Friary, incorporated into later buildings, but these are now demolished[7]. Traces of a mediaeval building were discovered during demolition adjacent to Johnny Ball Lane in 1989. The

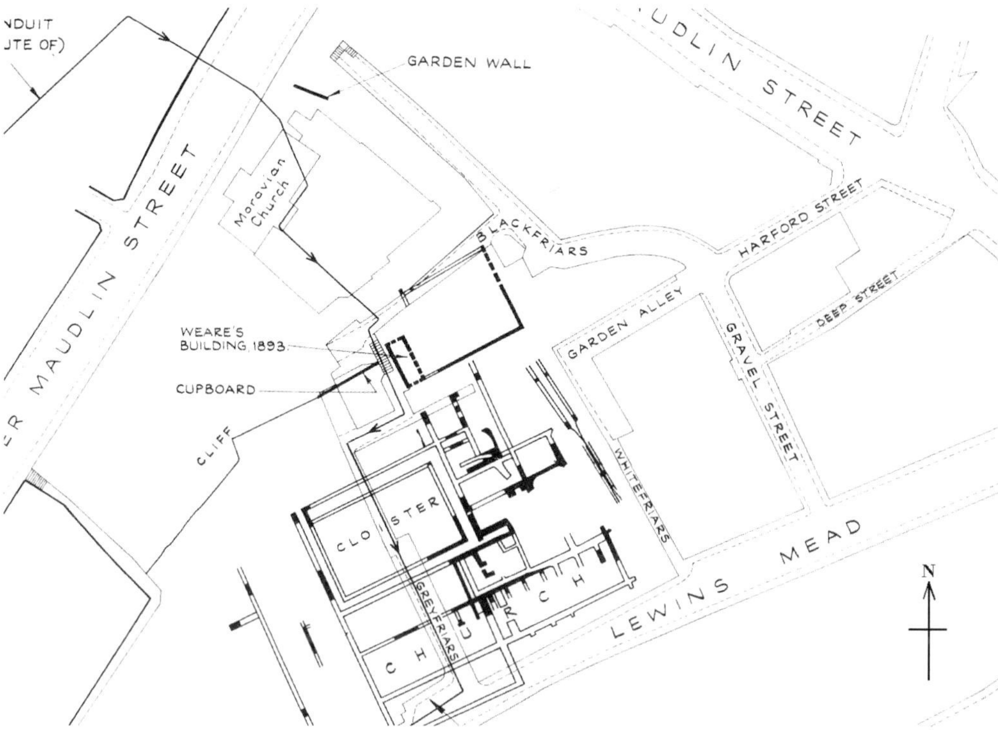

Figure 6. The plan of Greyfriars revealed by the 1973 excavation showing the line of the All Saints conduit (Copyright and courtesy of Bristol Museums, Galleries & Archives). The names Whitefriars and Blackfriars shown here are entirely without basis and seem to have been introduced erroneously in the 19th century.

present appropriately named Abbot's House, is now the headquarters of the BRI charity "Above and Beyond" (formerly the Special Trusttes of the United Bristol Hospitals). The new building contains a mediaeval beam and a small oval window incorporated from the earlier building[8].

The Moravians came to Bristol in the mid 18th century. They claimed descent from a Bohemian religious group which had reformed under the patronage of Count von Zinzendorf. Unlike other nonconformist groups they had no quarrel with the Church of England but wished to promote a more actively committed Christian life. Although a group had first worshipped together in Bristol as early as 1746 it was not until a visit by Count von Zinzendorf himself in 1755 that the congregation of about 50 became established. According to the Moravian Church Diary 1804 -1806 the brethren who had been living in temporary accommodation near Temple Street finally found a site for a permanent settlement in 1755. The described this as being "in Blackfriars, St James' Parish, a spot retired from the hurry and noise of the city" . The foundation stone for their chapel in what is now Upper Maudlin Street was laid on August 28th 1756 and the chapel was opened on June 25th 1757. The greater part of the cost had been borne by two only brethren, Thomas and Mortimer, as the majority of the congregation were poor[9].

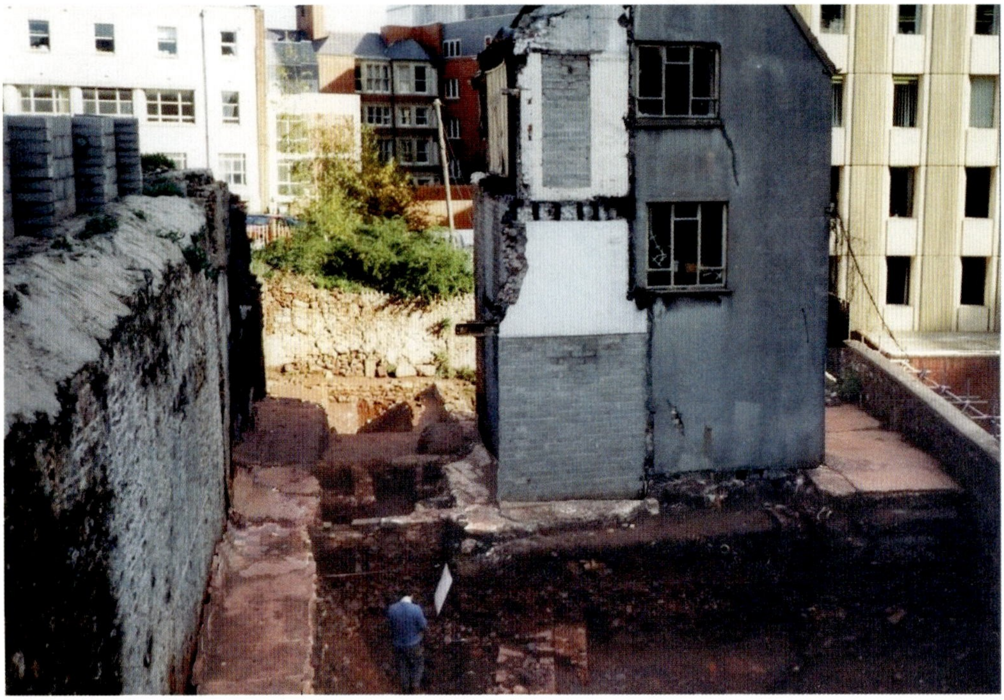

Figure 7a. The original Abbots House before demolition, looking NE towards the rear of the Dental School and Eye Hospital in1999.

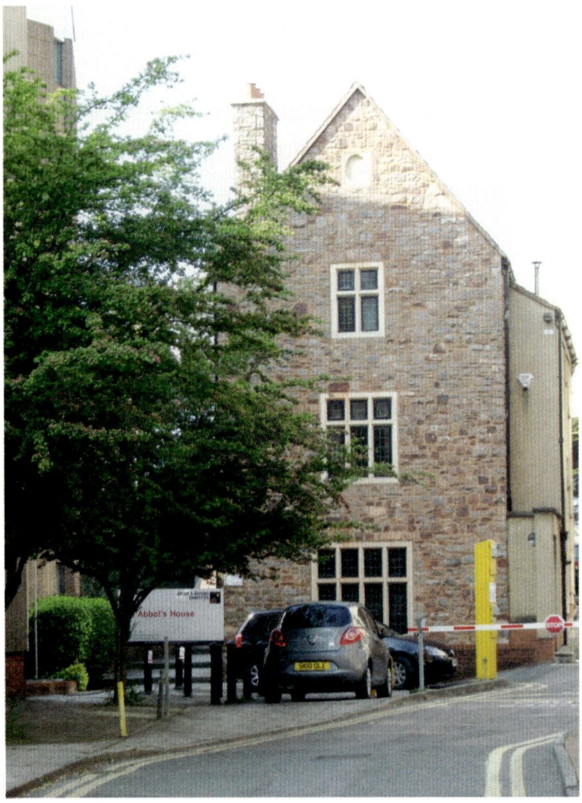

Figure 7b. The rebuilt Abbots House today looking SW.

According to Dresser[10] the Bristol Moravians or more correctly, "The Unity of the Brethren" never numbered more than 200. They shared much in common with the Quakers and Wesleyans but the Bristol Moravians were generally less affluent than Unitarian or Quakers in the city but had fewer poor and unskilled members than the Wesleyans The most prominent of the Moravian congregation were mainly small manufacturers but at least one, Samuel Fripp, was a partner of Fry, Fripp and Company who were engaged in exporting soap. Mortimer, mentioned above was, described as a "pin maker".

Sexual segregation was the cornerstone of their church's organisation. Their congregation was divided into "choirs" of single sisters, single brothers, married couples, widows, and widowers[11]. Single sisters and for a short while single brothers had a communal living and working space[12]. The sect also practised "oeconomy" where girls were taught an occupation. For these reasons shortly after acquiring their site on Upper Maudlin Street the Moravians entered into protracted negotiations to purchase an adjoining estate and a sisters house was established in an existing building on the site in June 1758. (This was improved and enlarged in 1764). It will be seen that their later premises includes a Sisters house and Brethren house for unmarried men and women, (Figure 15, 16).

Very little is known of the inner furnishings of the chapel apart from the contemporary sketch of 1907 shown in Figure 9. It is clear from the records of John Smith and Son's,

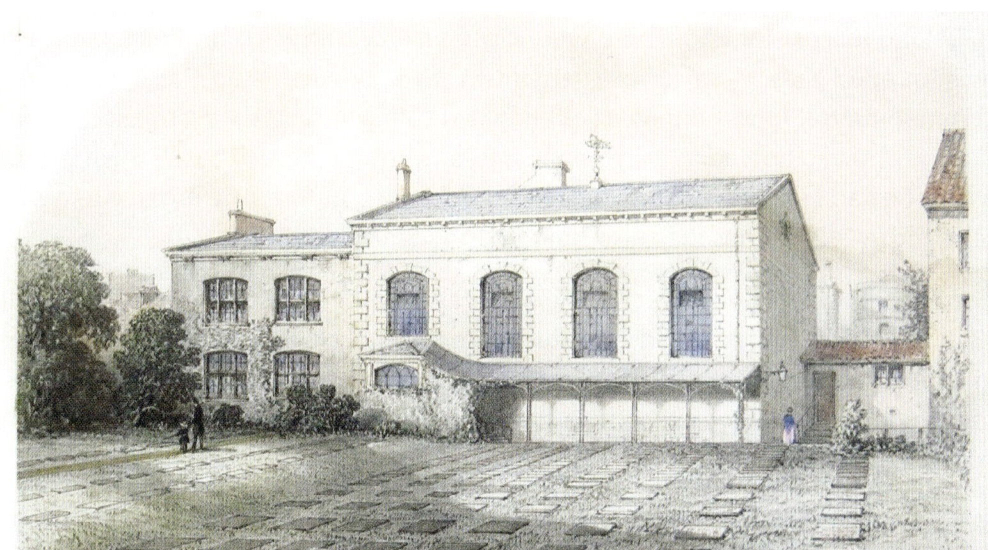

Figure 8. This later rear view of the Moravian Chapel shows the first school and Hall on the left and the passage leading to the Minister's House on the extreme right. In the foreground there are now a large number of graves with the gravestones laid flat and all the same size as was the Moravian custom.

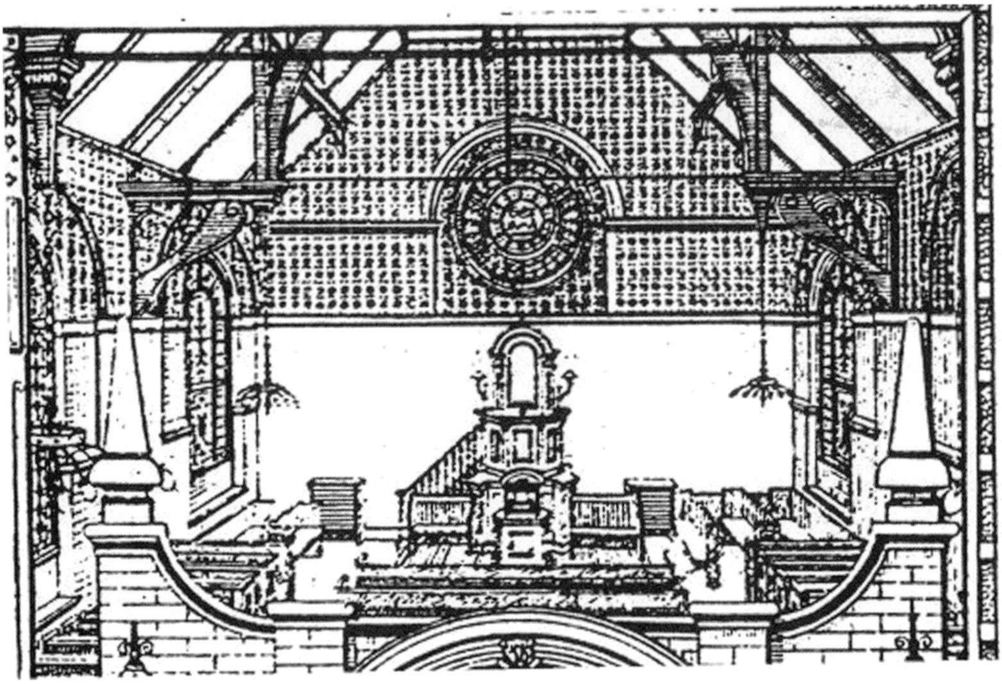

Figure 9. A contemporary sketch of the interior of the Moravian Chapel in 1907 looking towards the east window.

well known Bristol Organ Builders that it had an organ from its earliest days[13]. This is also reported as being a fine instrument in the Moravian Church Diary 1804-1806. The first organ was subsequently sold to the Moravian chapel at Gracehill, N. Ireland in 1781 for £30. There were close links with this community. Gracehill was founded as a Moravian settlement in 1765. A plaque on the church wall commemorates John Cennick (1718–1755) the first Moravian evangelist in mid Antrim who had arrived in Ballymena on 9 August 1746 from Kingswood in Bristol where he had established a Moravian Church 5 years before. The organ was again replaced in 1829 by another, also built by John Smith senior.

The chapel was long involved in the anti-slavery movement. On the 4th of April 1759, an African prince called *Gonglass* visited Maudlin Street, Bristol, and spoke in French to the minister there. It has been suggested that he was probably one of the sons of the powerful African slave trader John Currantee of Anamaboe, in present-day Ghana.

Mary Anne Schimmelpenninck née Galton (1778 – 1856), a prominent writer in the anti-slavery movement in Britain and aunt of Sir Francis Galton FRS, was buried in the chapel's graveyard. In 1806 Mary had married Lambert Schimmelpenninck, a Dutch shipping merchant, and moved from Birmingham to Bristol to be with him there. She died in Clifton and has a memorial tablet in the Cathedral. Another

Moravian family buried there were the descendants of Frederick James Badham[14] who followed the Moravian tradition of giving his children the surname of a prominent Moravian, as a middle name. Frederick died on the 15th April 1833 in Penzance but his body must have been brought back to Bristol, because his Moravian burial was recorded on the 23rd April of that year in the register of the Upper Maudlin Street chapel.

Bristol had grown rapidly in the 18th century. The population was probably about 25,000 in 1700. It rose to about 50,000 by the middle of the century. On the map of the city in 1773 (Figure 10) the only building shown between the Old Bristol Royal Infirmary (7) and Johnny Ball Lane is the Moravian chapel (19) with its burial ground at the rear. The Bristol Infirmary had opened in 1737 and by this time Marlborough Street had been constructed. This is named after John Churchill first Duke of Marlborough who had played a crucial role in the war of the Spanish succession and who had died in 1722. The land to the north of Maudlin Street appears by this time to have changed from the open fields of the 17th century to formal gardens. The Colston Alms houses (1691) can be seen on St. Michael's Hill as can the new Unitarian Chapel (18) built in 1787 on Lewins Mead.

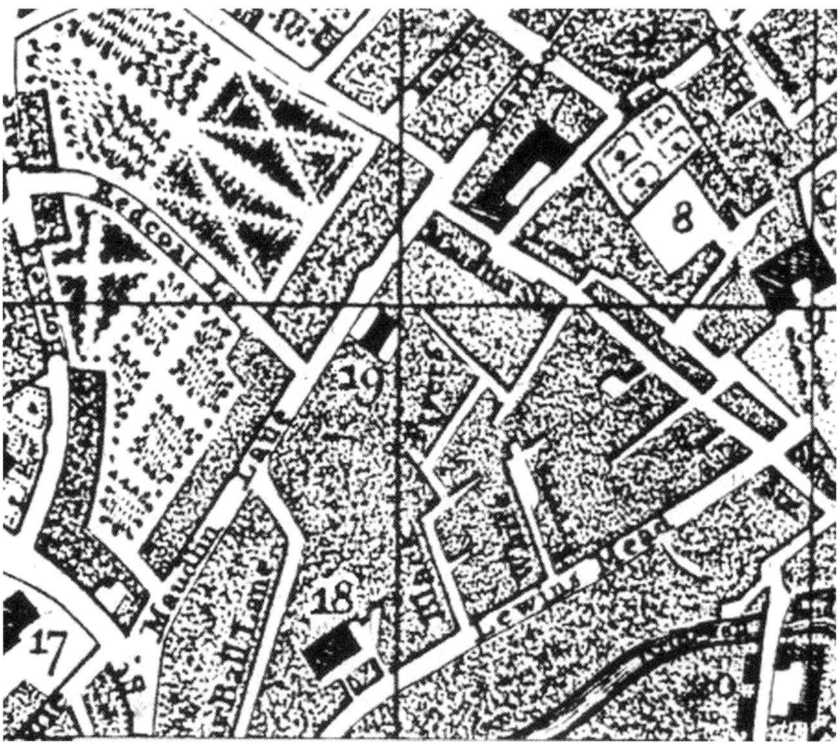

Figure 10. This map of 1773 still shows Upper Maudlin Street as Maudlin Lane. Its continuation, which would become Lower Maudlin Street, is shown as Maudlin Street.

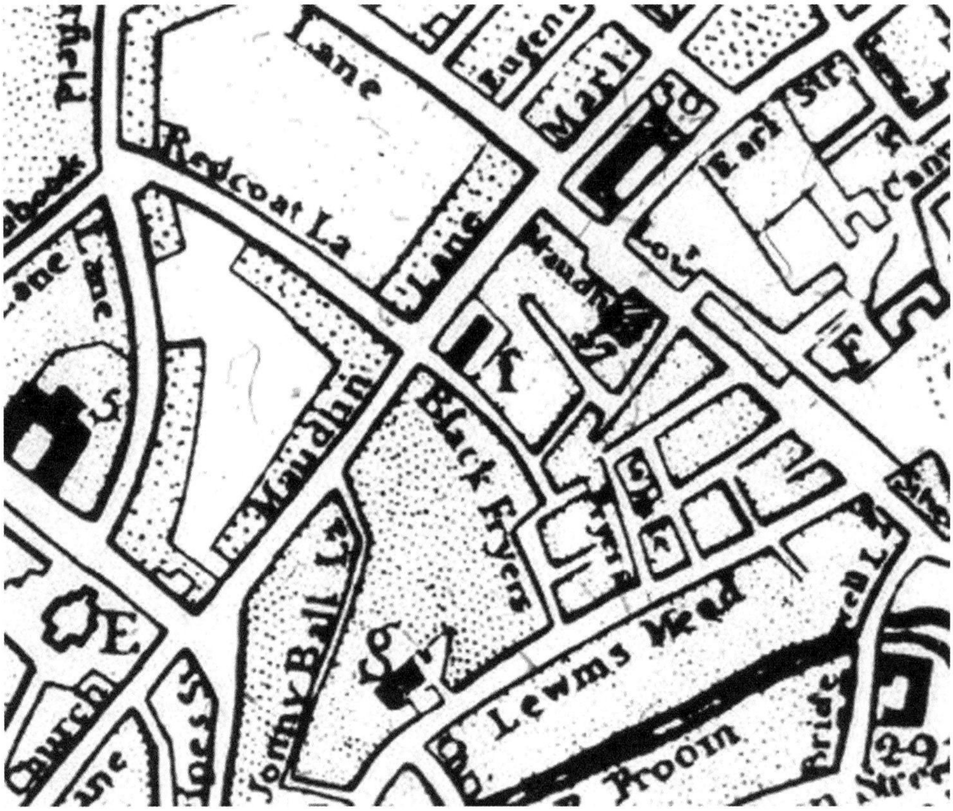

Figure 11. The map of 1815. f = Moravian Chapel; g = Unitarian Chapel. Curiously the Female Penitentiary which opened in 1801 is not shown.

By the late 18th century, the area of Kingsdown where formerly the King's cavalry had performed its daily drills was being developed as Bristol's first planned suburb. Up until this time the land which had once belonged to the Benedictine Priory of St James had been appreciated as an airy, green space just beyond the crowded medieval city. Some of the roads in which these houses were built, such as Redcoat Lane, disappeared during the subsequent development of the Royal Infirmary site (See Figure 11). At this time Upper and Lower Maudlin Streets appear under several different names[15]. The map of 1815 also shows that there is now an asylum for the blind on the site where the Eye Hospital stands today (marked as 37 in Figure 11) .This had been founded here in 1810 to give the blind the means of earning their own living. In June of that year, Dr William Henry Goldwyre, negotiated the rental of one house, number 12 Lower Maudlin Street, from the Blind Asylum and founded the Bristol Eye Hospital. The same building was bought from the Asylum in 1839 when the Asylum moved to Park Street[16]. This later building for the Bristol Asylum and School of Industry for the Blind occupied the site now taken up by the University's Wills Memorial Building and the City Museum and Art Gallery.

By 1828 a new building had appeared, near the corner of Maudlin Lane and Lower Maudlin Street – a female penitentiary marked as 35 in Figure 12; see also Figure 13. The penitentiary had been founded after a meeting on 23rd April 1801 in the vestry room of St. James' Barton which had considered "the possibility of affording an asylum to those unhappy females who have been seduced from the path of virtue and may be found desirous of returning into it". By this time the parishes of St James, St. Judes and St Michael's were identified as those having the highest number of brothels and the worst problems with prostitution in the city[17]. Subscribers were sought, a plan was circulated, and a Penitentiary was set up in Upper Maudlin Street with accommodation for about forty women. They were employed in such tasks as shoe-making, needlework and laundering and were later put into service. The time spent in the Penitentiary was usually up to one year but sometimes up to two. By this time St. James church was becoming overcrowded and in 1861 the Friends and Supporters of the Penitentiary formed a Committee to erect St. James-the-Less chapel[18]. This was designed by Pope & Bindon, well known architects of the time who were responsible for many Bristol buildings including the completion of Bristol Cathedral. The church was sited next to the penitentiary and had a distinctive domed east-end, termed a chevet. (See Figure 18 and 20). The opening service was held on 30th November 1867.

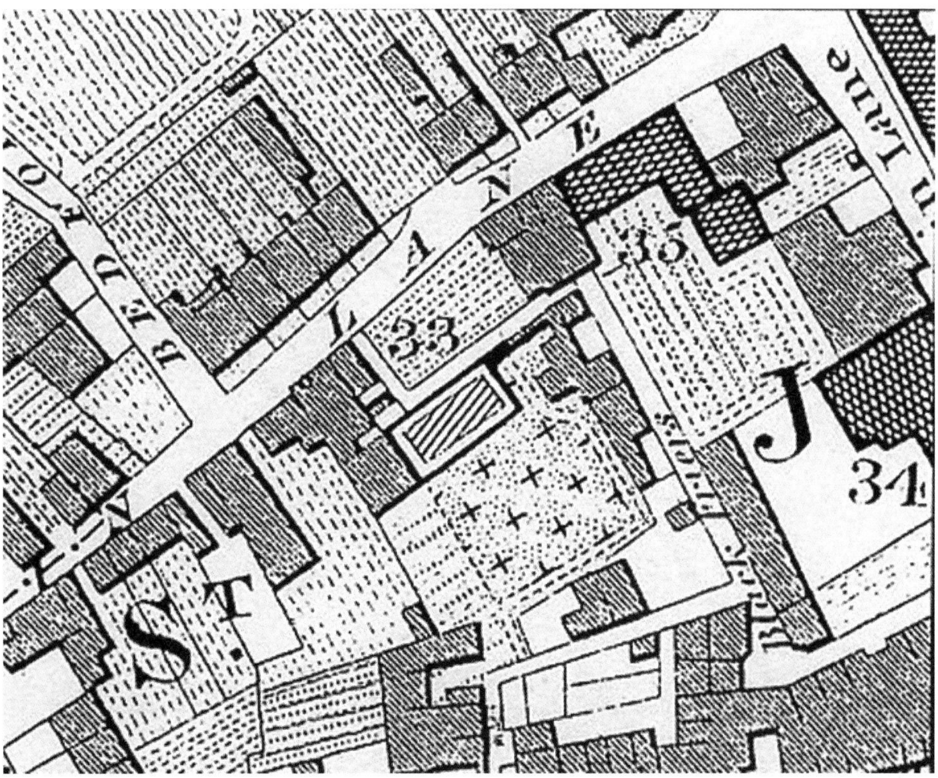

Figure 12. Ashmead's map of 1828. The Penitentiary building (35) was modified in the 1860s to allow the church of St James the less to be built, see Figures 10 and 11. Note also the relocation of the road named "Blackfriars".

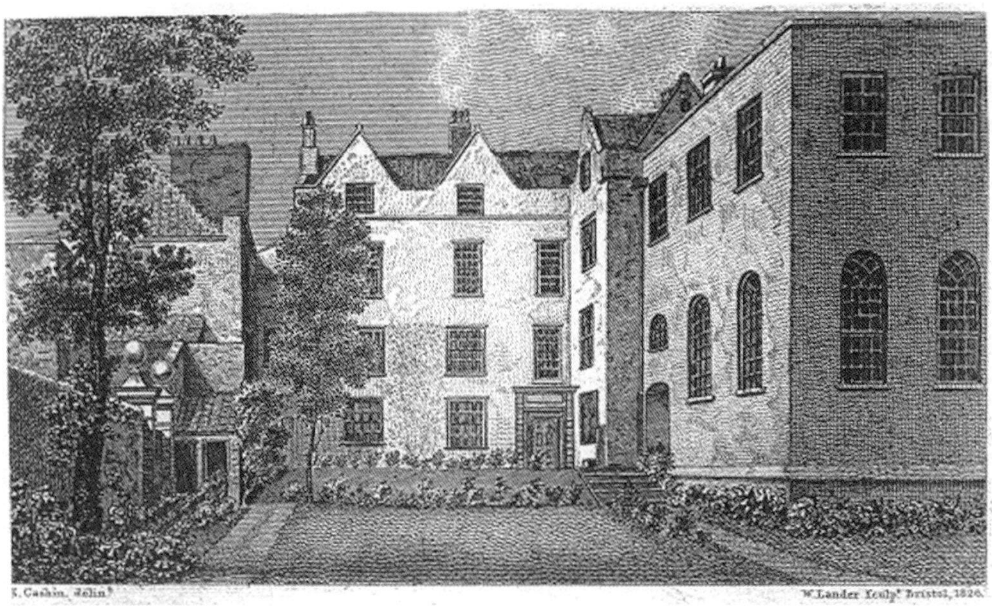

Figure 13. The Female Penitentiary view from inside the yard shown on the map in Figure 9. The road, now named Blackfriars, is beyond the wall on the left. The building facing was demolished to allow the St James the less to be built.

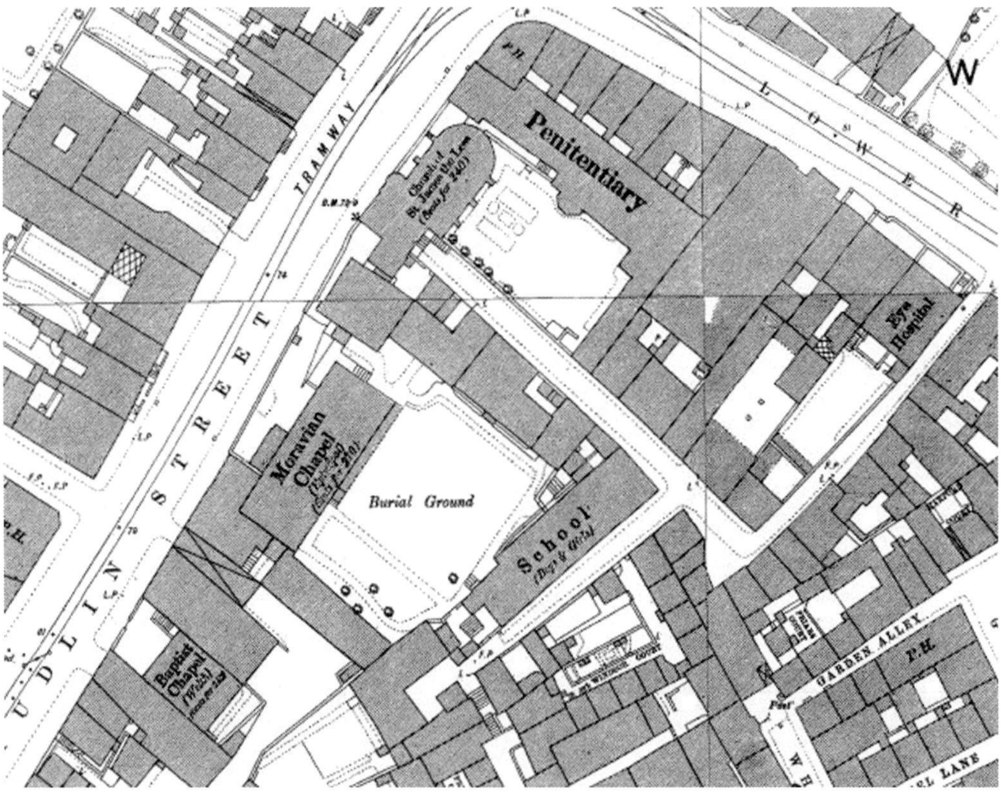

Figure 14. The map of 1884.

The map of 1884 (Figure 14) shows other new developments. Shops had been built between the Female Penitentiary and the Eye Hospital in what is today's Lower Maudlin Street. The corner site of Upper and Lower Maudlin Streets had become a public house - The Prince Alfred - which would remain there until its demolition in the 1960s to make way for the dental school's 1964 extension. Route 3 of the Bristol Tramways Company ran along Upper and Lower Mudlin Street. Horse drawn trams had been introduced 10 years earlier. The arched entrance of the present "Zero Degrees" gastro-pub at the junction of Perry Road and Colston Street was formerly the entrance to the horsedrawn tram depot and its stables. In 1895 Bristol would become the first city to adopt electric trams. These continued to run until the Luftwaffe's Good Friday bombing raid of 1941 destroyed the company's generating station.

Like so many nonconformists the Moravians had their school adjacent to the chapel. By 1870 there is also a separate girls' school shown on the plan (Figure 15). This is probably because the Moravians had from their earliest days separated the sexes and by 1828, 68% of their congregation were women. The chapel and its buildings were still located in an area of light industry. There was a cooperage on the corner of Lower

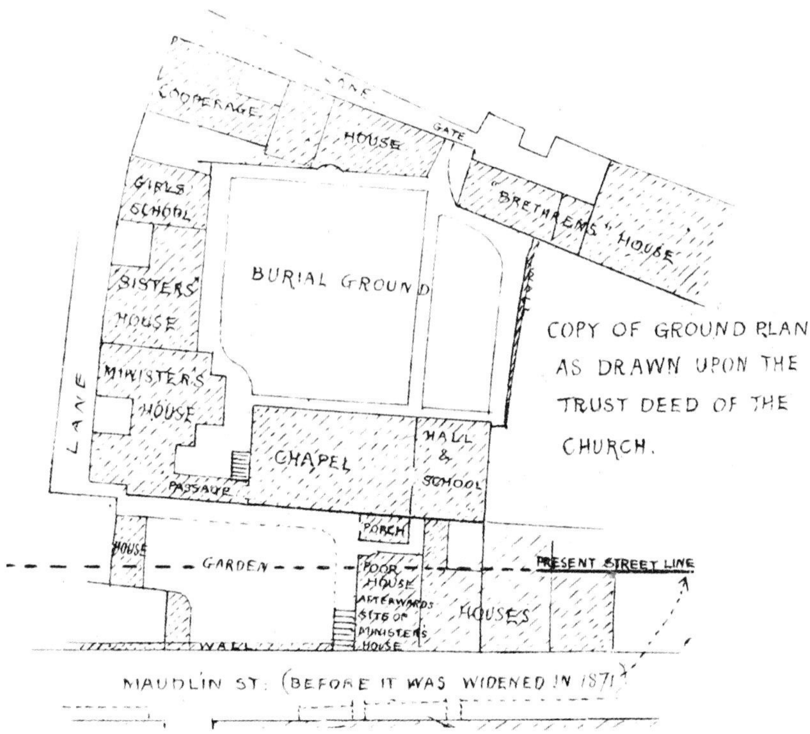

Figure 15. The site of the Moravian chapel as it was in 1870 before the widening of Upper Maudlin Street in 1871*

* From "A short sketch of the work carried out by the Ancient Protestant Episcopal Church ,1887" by kind permission of Special Collections of Bristol University.

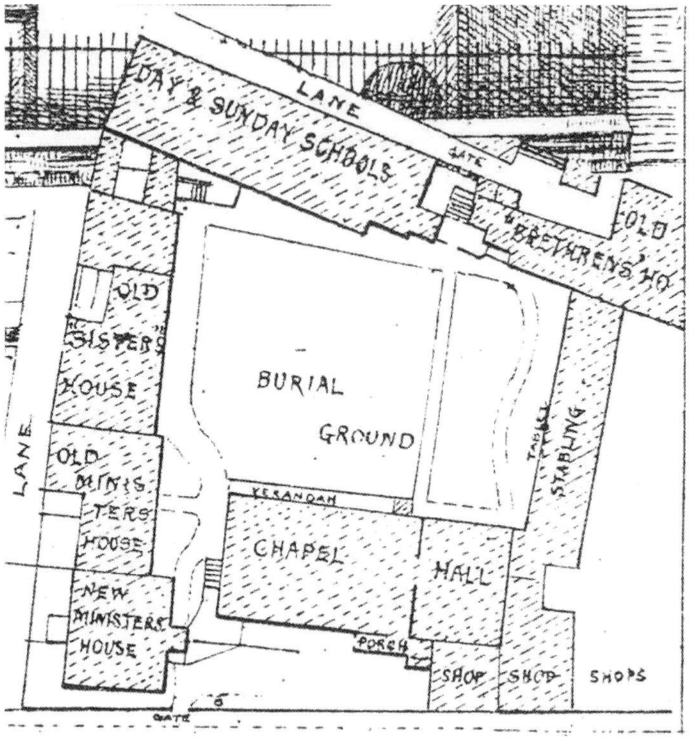

Figure 16. The Moravian chapel site in 1887 after building revisions. *

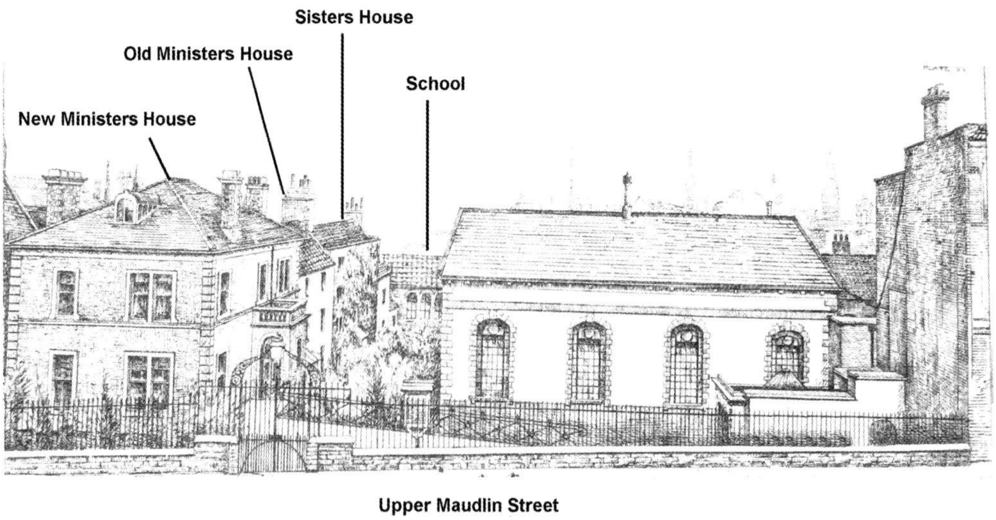

Figure 17. Looking south into Moravian Place from Upper Maudlin Street c. 1890. *

---

* From "A short sketch of the work carried out by the Ancient Protestant Episcopal Church, 1887" by kind permission of Special Collections of Bristol University.

Maudlin Street, although whether this was run by a member of the sect is unknown. The area was not prosperous as indicated by the chapel's close proximity to the Poor House before it was lost to road widening (Figure 15).

By 1887 the Moravian Chapel had been modified and a new minister's house constructed beside it (Figures 16, 17). The narrow road leading past these buildings from Upper Maudlin Street to the burial ground was called Moravian Place. To the south of the burial ground the cooperage and the cooper's house have been replaced by an enlarged school and Sunday school (Figure.11). A hostel for retired Moravian ministers was adjacent to this. Further shops had opened fronting Upper Maudlin Street between the Moravian chapel and Johnny Ball Lane but it is not clear if the stabling was part of the Moravian property.

A member of the congregation at this time was James Fuller Eberle (1854-1939) who was married there in 1880. He had been a school fellow of George Alfred and Henry Hubert Wills and was in turn Alderman and later Freeman of the City as well as founder and first honorary member of Clifton Rugby Club. He also saved the Elizabethan Bristol Red Lodge from demolition and gave it to the city. He held the Order of the Russian Red Cross and was an officer of the Order of the British Empire.

The map of 1903 (Figure 18) shows very clearly the former buildings on the dental school site which are reflected in the outlines of today's buildings. The Penitentiary closed in 1891 and was sold in 1899 to become a brass foundry. There was little change in the area from this time until building started for the new Dental School.

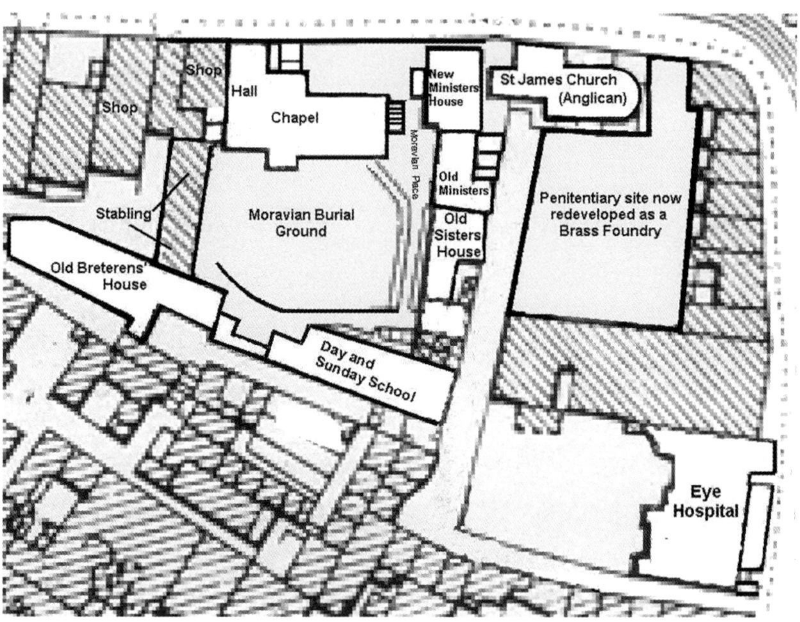

Figure 18. The area of the Dental School site redrawn from the map of 1903.

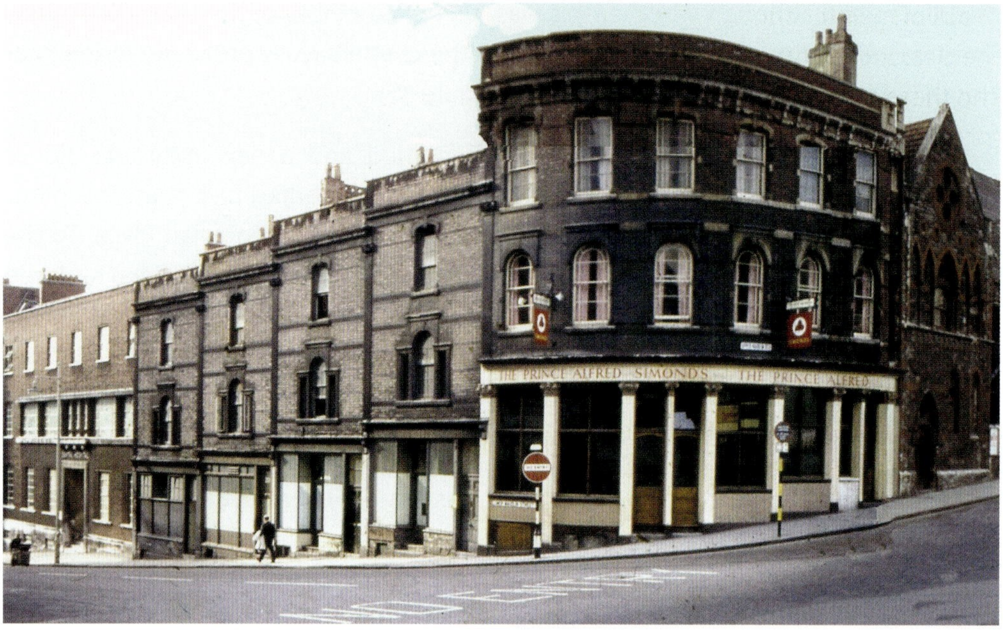

Figure 19. The corner of Upper and Lower Maudlin Streets in 1960.

By 1939 the Dental School and Hospital had been completed, its frontage replacing two of the shops in Lower Maudlin Street. The appearance of the street remained as shown in Figure 20 until the remaining four shops, including the tea shop run by Mrs Room and the Prince Alfred pub, were demolished to make way for the 1964 extension.

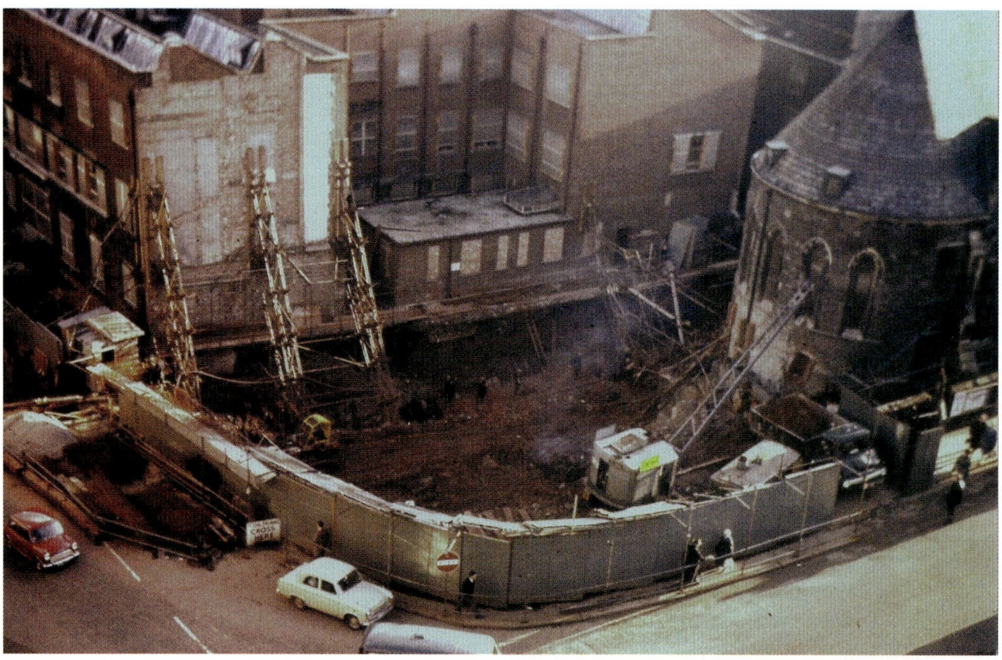

Figure 20. The same corner as Figure 19 in 1963, after clearance ready for the 1964 extension.

A lack of maintenance, coupled with Second World War damage would soon result in the clearance of other houses of a similar vintage to the north of Upper Maudlin Street and these sites and the Kingsdown slopes behind them were, by this time, earmarked for hospital expansion and municipal housing[19].

The outline of the brass foundry is recorded on the 1953 Ordnance Survey map but its use is unmarked. The photograph in Figure 21 shows this building just prior to its demolition in 1962 and is the rear view of the buildings shown in Figure 19. The tall chimney in the background still exists as part of the old BRI building on the far side of Lower Maudlin Street. The first buttress of the former church of St James the less is just visible on the extreme left of the picture . The church had closed by this time and was being used by the Church Lads Brigade. It was also serving as a venereal disease clinic for the Bristol Royal Infirmary until this could be relocated when the Royal Infirmary's Queens building opened.

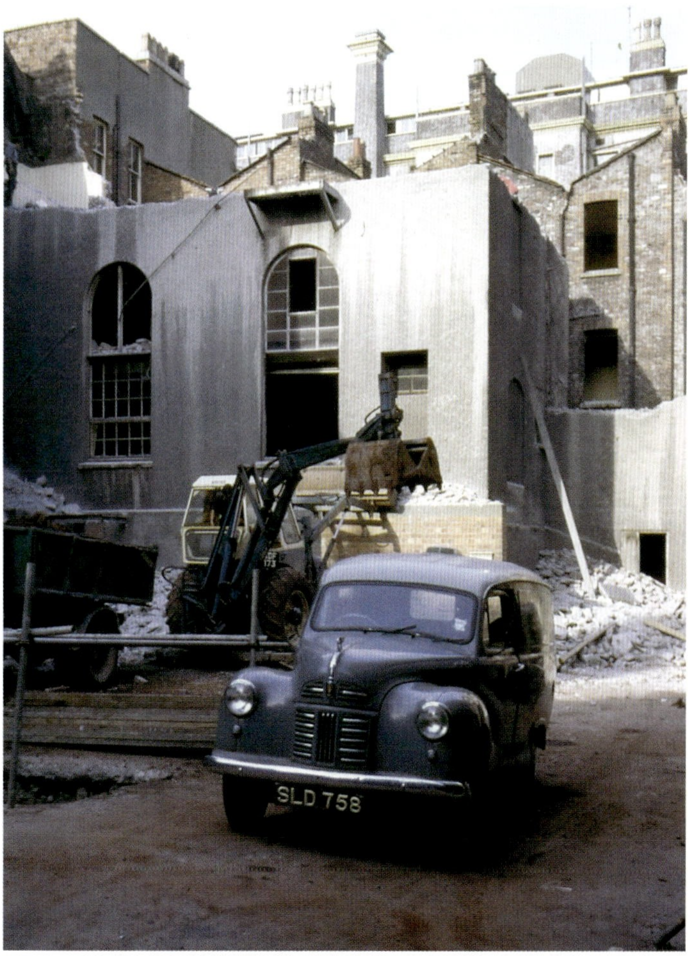

Figure 21. The rear view of the buildings shown in Figure 19.

The map in Figure 22 shows the site in about 1970 with the chevet of St James the less left almost touching the side of the new building. The school and Sunday school buildings beyond the Moravian Burial Ground, still existed as a paint works at this time. The Moravian church itself closed in 1971 the closing service being held at 3:00pm on Saturday 31st July of that year[20].

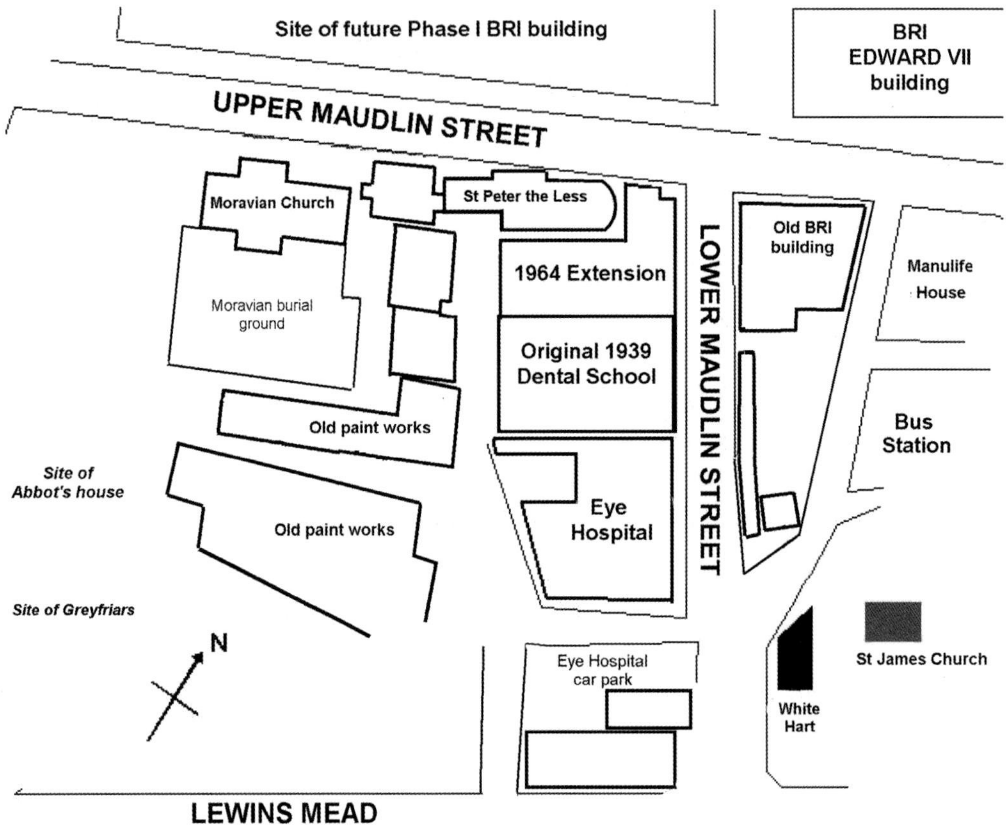

Figure 22. The key buildings of the site in about 1970 (not to scale).

The second extension of the Dental School took place in 1973, after demolition of the Moravian Chapel, St. James the Less church and adjacent buildings. It was built on the site of St James the less to provide staff offices and research laboratories for the MRC Dental Research Unit. Originally funded by the Wellcome Foundation it is still known as the Wellcome Building.

A third extension to the School was opened in 1984 and was built on the site of the Moravian chapel. It was preceded by extensive archaeological investigations of the site. When completed the 1984 building provided a much needed new operative dental techniques laboratory, an extended and modernised dental library plus a dental materials laboratory.

The most recent extension, known as the Chapter House, was completed in 1995. It was built on the site of the former burial ground of the Moravian Chapel and the long demolished paint works. The building was officially opened by Her Majesty the Queen in June of that year. Because so much University space in the original building had been taken up by clinical facilities, the Chapter house reprovided this much need research, tutorial and office space. As the Chief Executive at the time remarked "It is only occasion I have heard of where NHS funds have been used to provide a University Building!"

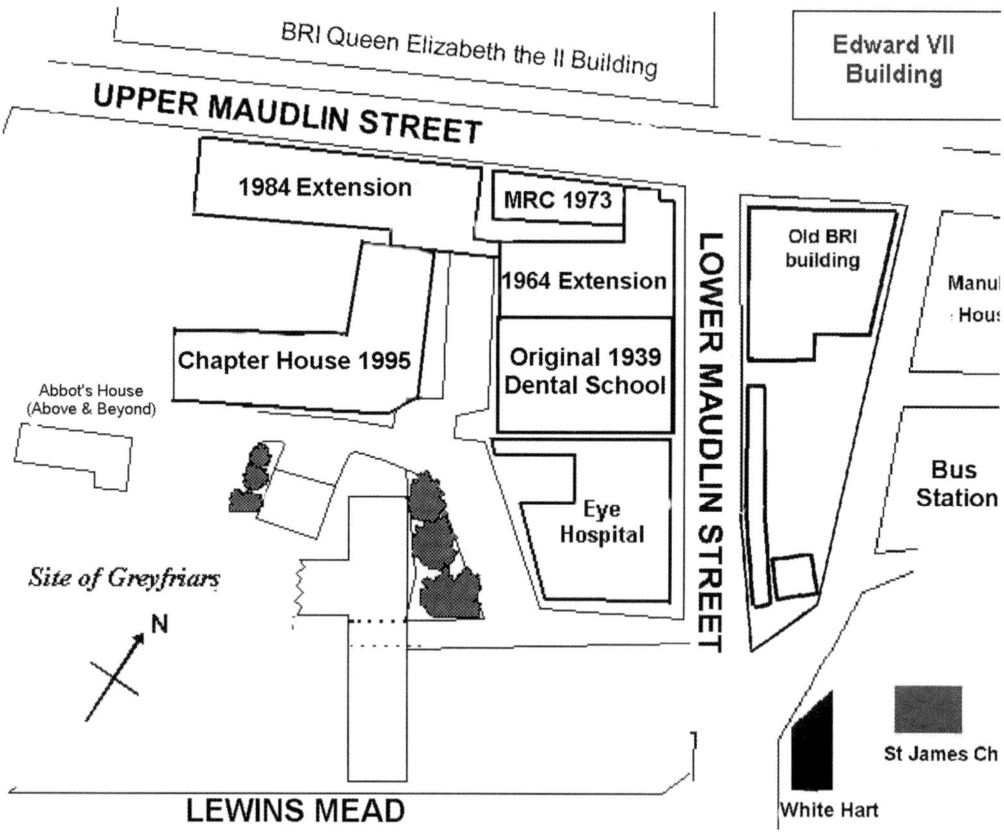

Figure 23. The site today (2012).

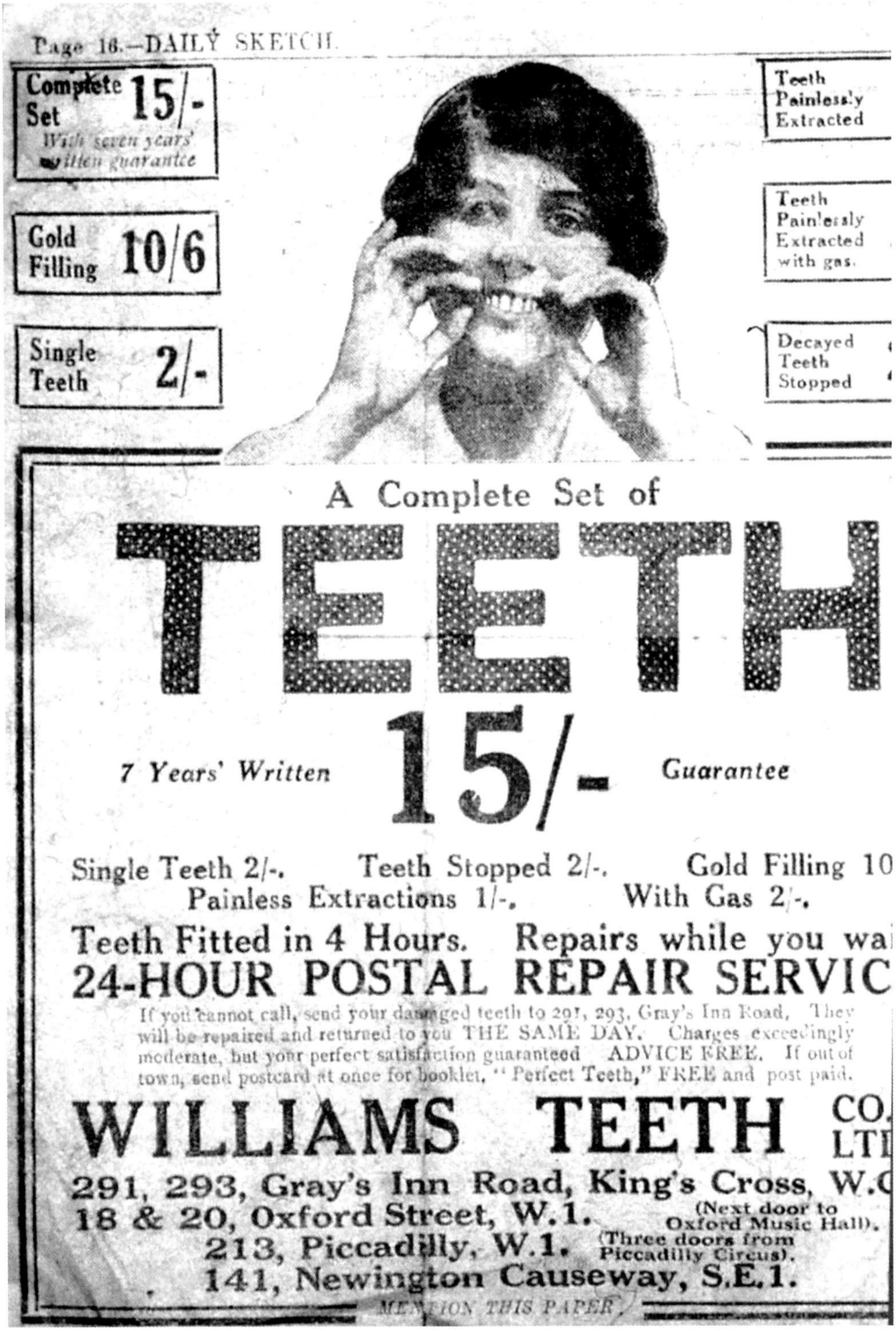

Figure 24. An advertisement of unregistered late 19th century dentist getting round the problem of avoiding the title "dentist" or "dental surgeon".

Chapter 2

THE EVOLUTION OF THE DENTAL PROFESSION IN BRITAIN

Dentistry, of a sort, has been practised for many thousands of years. The first written account of any value was that contained in *Book VII Chapter 12* of *Celsus* great work *De Medicina* of about AD 50. Written in Latin this was one of the first books to be printed. The first English text was *The Operator of the Teeth* by Charles Allen published in 1685[21] and *Celsus' De Medicina* and several other texts on dentistry had been translated into English by the early 19th century.

Despite this 19th century dentistry was still a "trade" practised by three groups. By far the largest was a group of uneducated and unqualified persons who attracted clients by blatant advertising. Some of these also saw the provision of training as a useful income stream and offered short courses lasting from a few days to a few months claiming to provide "all the skills necessary to undertake the duties of a dentist"[22].

Next there were a group of those who had been pupils (apprentices) to dentists, usually of good local reputation, for three to five years. A. J. Woodhouse (1824-1906), gives a clear picture of his own apprenticeship in Exeter the 1840's as follows:

> *"I had the good fortune to be placed with Mr. Thomas Sheffield of Exeter, who was in the forefront of the best practitioners of his day... My articles bound me to Mr. Sheffield for four years, in them he undertook to teach me ' the art, mystery, and professional employment of a dentist', and I promised to 'serve him faithfully and keep his secrets'. The mode of instructing me that Mr. Sheffield adopted was to work with me at the bench and occasionally to take me into his surgery, where I saw him operate. I was also at his side when he saw the gratis patients who came to him each morning at nine o'clock to be relieved of pain. I did all his mechanical work during my apprenticeship, and after about three months he gave the care of the gratis patients into my hands, and I well remember when I went down alone to extract my first tooth, which I am happy to say I accomplished successfully. From that time I selected from among the cleanest of these poor people those who needed teeth stopped, and attended to them. Mr. Sheffield used to examine the teeth when I had prepared them,*

and afterwards when the filling was completed, but he soon left me to my own devices, except when any great difficulty arose, when he always came to my help. After about a year or so, he left me in charge of his private patients when he went for his holiday... We, at Exeter, made most of our own instruments, for those to be bought were very indifferent; we even made our own forceps, carefully adjusting them to the teeth for which they were to be used. . . . In my early days we got our gold leaf and tin from local gold-beaters. ... I had sometimes to go to their workshop and wait while it was beaten..."[23]

In Bristol Mr. W. R. Ackland of 5 Rodney Place, Clifton had two paying pupils at any one time who stayed for two years and perhaps four apprentices who were contracted to stay a longer period of up to five years, with remuneration as they became more efficient.

Finally there was a small elite group of educated men who had medical or surgical qualifications and who chose to practise dental surgery. Although earlier efforts had been made to reform marketplace dentistry it was not until 1858 that the provisions of the Medical Act allowed the Royal College of Surgeons of England to institute the Licentiate in Dental Surgery. In the same year the Dental Hospital of London opened, the first clinical training establishment for dentists in Britain.

1. That it shall be lawful for the Council of the said College to appoint a Board of Examiners for the purpose of testing the fitness of persons to practise as Dentists who may be desirous of being so examined, and to grant Certificates of such fitness. And it is our will and pleasure that such Board of Examiners be called the Board of Examiners in Dental Surgery, and consist of not less than six Members, to be appointed as hereinafter mentioned, three of whom shall be Members of the Court of Examiners for the time being of the said College, and the others of them shall be such persons skilled in Dental Surgery as the Council of the said College shall from time to time think proper to appoint.

1. Power of Council to appoint a Board of Examiners for testing the fitness of persons to practise as Dentists, and to grant Certificates of such fitness.
That such Board consist of not less than 6 Members, 3 to be Members of the Court of Examiners of the College, and the others to be persons skilled in Dental Surgery.

Figure 25. An extract from the Medical Act of 1858.

The first LDS examination was held by the College in London in 1860 with 60 candidates. Despite this there was still no compulsion for dentists to hold such a qualification but the pressure for dental reform continued to grow. This culminated in the passing of the Dentists Act of 1878 (closely following the invention of the foot treadle engine by James Beall Morrison). From that date no person practising dentistry could describe themselves as a dentist, dental practitioner or any name title or description that implied this unless they were registered on a Dentists Register held by the General Medical Council. It will however be seen from the advertisement

(Figure 24) that it was not difficult to get round this limitation! Nevertheless there was a great rush to register which rather overwhelmed the GMC and this was soon followed by the establishment of the British Dental Association in the following year largely to monitor and offer comment on the working if the Act.

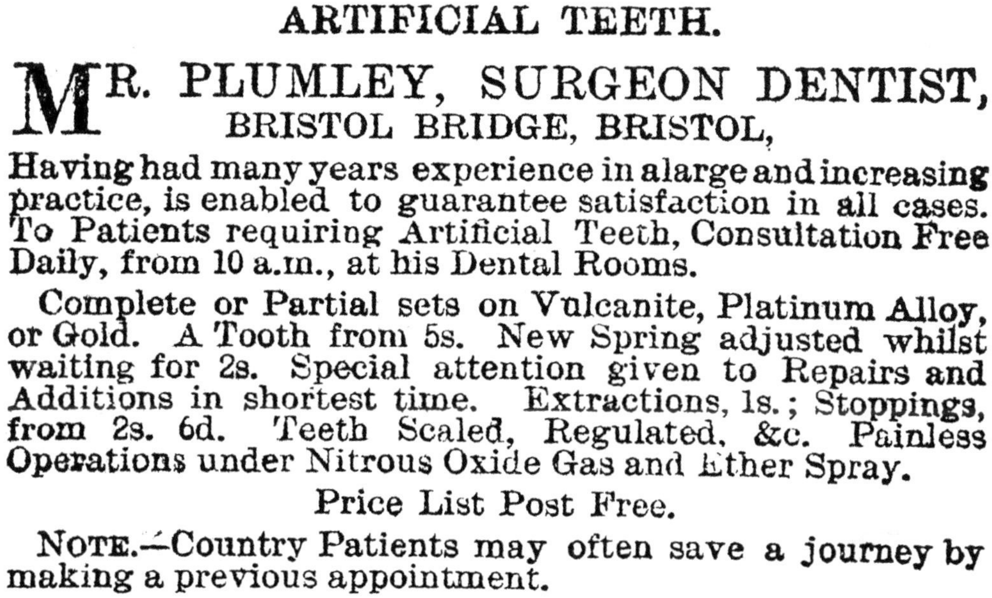

ARTIFICIAL TEETH.

MR. PLUMLEY, SURGEON DENTIST, BRISTOL BRIDGE, BRISTOL,

Having had many years experience in alarge and increasing practice, is enabled to guarantee satisfaction in all cases. To Patients requiring Artificial Teeth, Consultation Free Daily, from 10 a.m., at his Dental Rooms.

Complete or Partial sets on Vulcanite, Platinum Alloy, or Gold. A Tooth from 5s. New Spring adjusted whilst waiting for 2s. Special attention given to Repairs and Additions in shortest time. Extractions, 1s.; Stoppings, from 2s. 6d. Teeth Scaled, Regulated, &c. Painless Operations under Nitrous Oxide Gas and Ether Spray.

Price List Post Free.

NOTE.—Country Patients may often save a journey by making a previous appointment.

Figure 26. An advertisement from Bristol Times and Mirror of 7th January 1886. The title of "surgeon dentist" shows he has taken the LDSRCS.

It was not until the Dentists Act of 1921 that a dental (or medical) qualification was required for the practice of dentistry. Under this dentistry became regulated by a Dental Board but their recommendations required the approval of the General Medical Council. By this time all the Royal Colleges of Surgeons and many universities were offering dental qualifications - the first BDS degree was awarded by the University of Birmingham in 1901. All were recognised as licensing agencies by the GMC's Dental Board and these degrees and diplomas and the bodies which had awarded them were indicated in the Dentists Register. There was the need in 1921 to grandfather in all those unqualified persons who hitherto had been practising dentistry and as late as 1964 there were still on thousand unqualified persons listed in the Dentists Register as "Dentists Act, 1921".

Even so not all parties were happy with the new arrangements designed to bring dentistry under the medical administrative umbrella.

In 1956 the Dental Board of the General Medical Council was superseded by the General Dental Council at which point dentistry became a self regulating profession

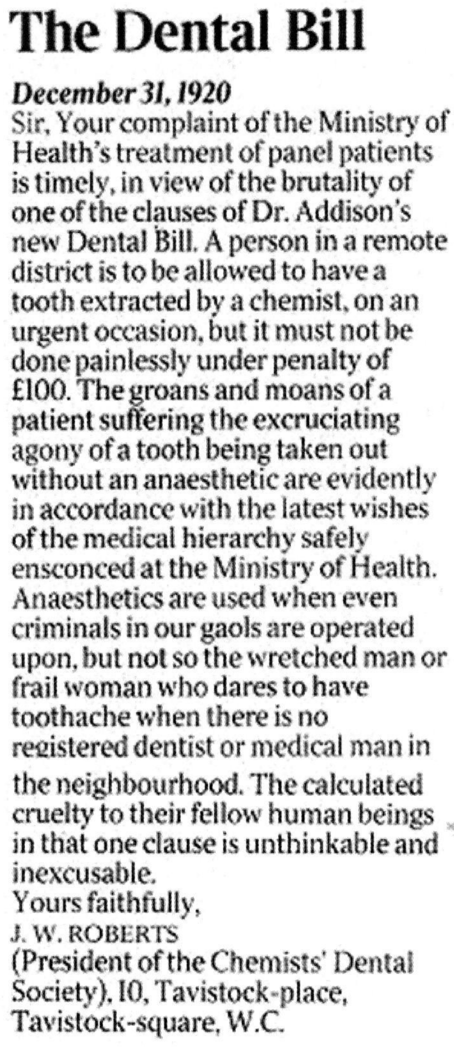
The Dental Bill

December 31, 1920

Sir, Your complaint of the Ministry of Health's treatment of panel patients is timely, in view of the brutality of one of the clauses of Dr. Addison's new Dental Bill. A person in a remote district is to be allowed to have a tooth extracted by a chemist, on an urgent occasion, but it must not be done painlessly under penalty of £100. The groans and moans of a patient suffering the excruciating agony of a tooth being taken out without an anaesthetic are evidently in accordance with the latest wishes of the medical hierarchy safely ensconced at the Ministry of Health. Anaesthetics are used when even criminals in our gaols are operated upon, but not so the wretched man or frail woman who dares to have toothache when there is no registered dentist or medical man in the neighbourhood. The calculated cruelty to their fellow human beings in that one clause is unthinkable and inexcusable.

Yours faithfully,

J. W. ROBERTS

(President of the Chemists' Dental Society), 10, Tavistock-place, Tavistock-square, W.C.

Figure 27. A letter to The Times from the president of the Chemists Dental Society.

although doctors were still permitted to practice dentistry. Finally in the 1984 Dentists Act the practise of dentistry by those holding a medical qualification was outlawed.

Chapter 3

THE ORIGINS OF DENTAL TEACHING IN BRISTOL

The origins of the Bristol Dental School can be found in three different institutions, the Bristol General Hospital, the Bristol Infirmary (later the Royal Infirmary), and the old University College which was eventually to become the University of Bristol. The Bristol Infirmary opened in 1736 with over 100 paid up subscribers which were of two classes. In the first class there was a life subscription of 30 guineas (equivalent to a curate's annual pay!) or you could pay 2 guineas annually. In the second there was a 15 guinea life subscription or payment of 1 guinea annually. Your guineas gave you patronage. Subscribers recommended the patients to be admitted and also had the choice of honorary medical staff.

To be elected an honorary physician or surgeon was a mark of great distinction. The apothecary had apprentices indentured for 7 years who were kept very busy by the honorary physicians. In their final year apprentices were allowed to become the pupil of a surgeon. Private pupils lived in the surgeon's house and paid handsomely for it. This was a significant source of income for the honorary surgeon. The more lowly "surgical pupils" were attached to all the visiting surgeons and paid a fee to the hospital. The Infirmary opened in June 1737 and soon had over 700 patients under treatment.

It was said that the Infirmary was Tory and Church, and also too small, and so in 1832 the Nonconformists and Liberals opened their own hospital, the Bristol General Hospital, and there was thereafter intense rivalry between the staff of the two hospitals.

The earliest recorded lectures given by Infirmary staff were those delivered in the Surgeons Hall by John Page and James Ford in 1746.[24] Lectures to the public by physicians, surgeons and "anatomists" also were commonplace and lectures to the public are recorded as early as 1785. Lectures in surgery were being given to students of the Infirmary by 1794. During the next thirty years such lectures became more frequent until by 1831 there were regular well attended courses of 60 lectures on the "Principles, practice and operations of surgery" given in the Infirmary museum by William Hetling.

The Bristol Medical School issued its first prospectus in 1832 and started the following year above a house in Park Row. It was an amalgamation of the 'Bristol Medical and Surgical School' and the 'School of Anatomy and Medicine'. With the Anatomy Act receiving the Royal assent in 1832 the days of the body snatching "anatomists" were over! The teaching of medicine and surgery thus preceded both the establishment of the University College (1876) and the passing of the first Dentists Act (1878). Medical students would "walk the wards" at either the Infirmary of the General Hospital. Dentistry at this time was seen to be part of surgery but in due course students could attend the dental departments of either the Bristol Infirmary or the Bristol General Hospital.

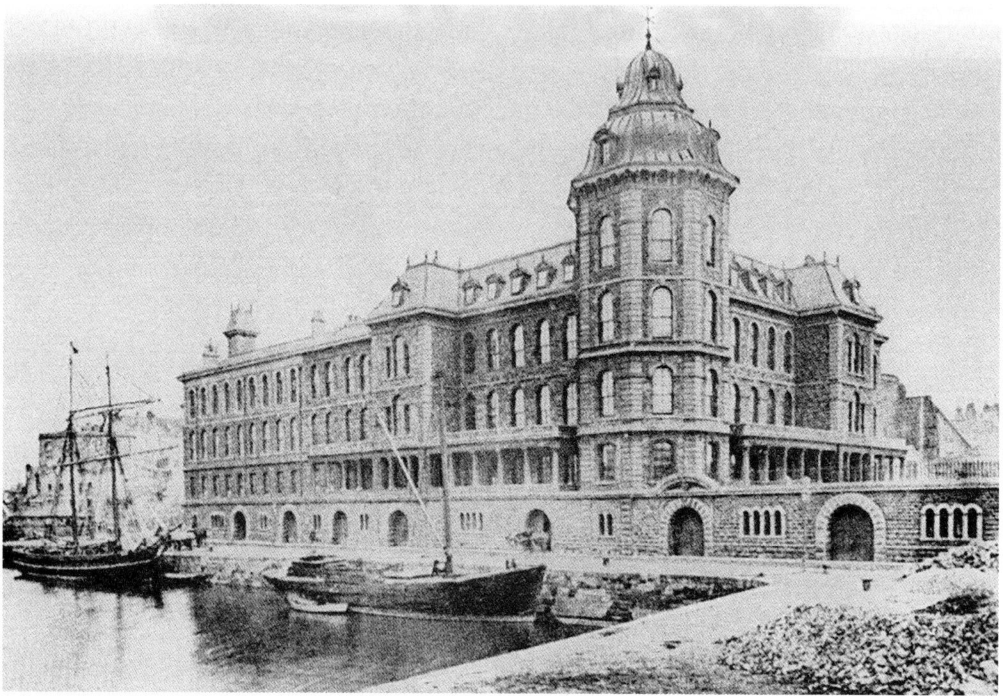

Figure 28. The Bristol General Hospital in about 1890.

The Bristol General Hospital had been the first to establish a post specific to dentistry[25] when in 1874 the position of surgeon dentist was created and Thomas Cooke Parsons elected to it. Dental duties up to that time had been performed by John H B Thwaites, but his official standing is not clear. Later, in 1880, the General Hospital was the first to establish a Department of dental surgery.

The Infirmary continued to expect dental procedures to be part of the duties of the general surgeon until 1888 when William Robert Ackland was appointed as their Dental Surgeon. It established its Dental Department in January 1888. This was the third of the three specialist departments which had been recommended by its Trustees in May 1885. Ackland had passed his LDSRCS in 1884 when he gave his address as Exeter. Before he came to Bristol, at the age of 25, he had been Demonstrator of Practical Dental Surgery at the London Dental Hospital, and Assistant Dental Surgeon at Charing Cross. He was to remain in his Bristol post until 1922. In March 1902 Charles. Hayman was appointed Honorary Dental Assistant "to instruct students in dental mechanics". Conditions in those days were still very primitive. Munro Smith, himself an assistant surgeon and then surgeon from 1889-1907 says in his history of the Bristol Royal Infirmary:

> *"The advantage of having a properly equipped department with expert dentists, and the many accessories necessary for tooth extraction, etc., was at once apparent, and the shrieks associated with this branch of surgery became confined to certain days".*[26]

The work of the Department grew rapidly necessitating a number of changes in the layout of Infirmary's outpatient department. By 1904 these changes had provided a dental operation room and greater space in the outpatients waiting room. On April 26th 1904 Dr. Hayman was appointed Assistant Dental Surgeon (one assumes that this meant he was now paid) and on April 11th 1905 Dr. Leonard A Moore was elected Honorary Anaesthetist of the Dental Department. Before this time the giving of anaesthetics had been part of the duties of the Resident Casualty Officer!

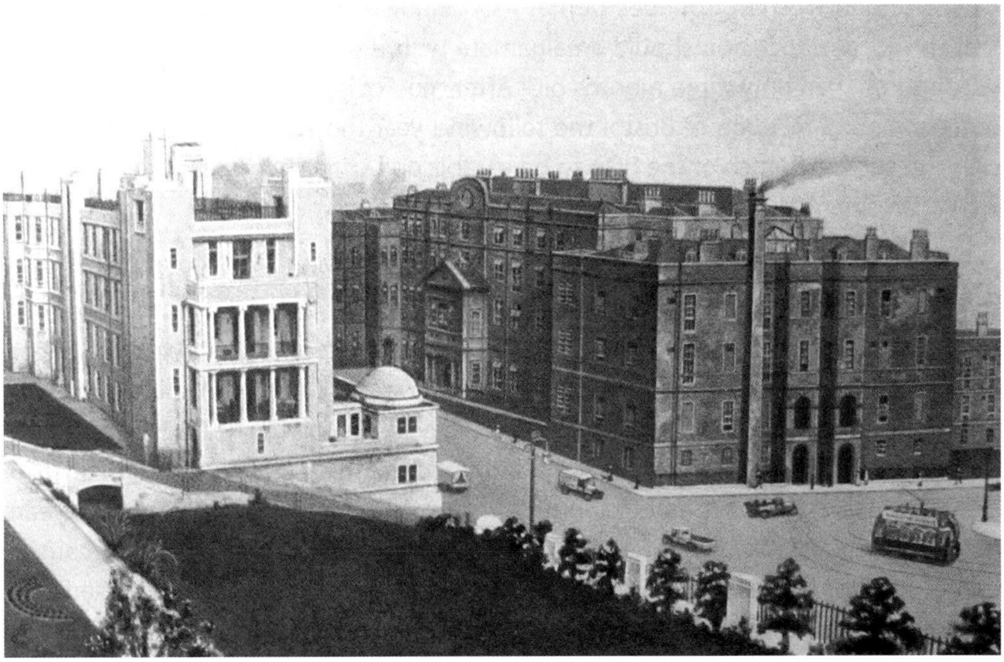

Figure 29. The Bristol Royal Infirmary in 1912 as Hayman would have known it.

Chapter 4

FROM COLLEGE TO UNIVERSITY

By 1870 there was already a movement among staff of the Bristol General Hospital and the Infirmary to establish a college of science and literature in the West of England and in June 1874 a meeting took place in the Victoria Rooms to promote a school of science and literature in the West of England. This cause was adopted by Dr Percival, (Headmaster of Clifton College and later Bishop of Hereford) who was supported by Jowett, Master of Balliol College Oxford, a major figure of the time. This became translated into a movement to establish a University College. In August 1876 the first meeting of the College Council was held under the Chairmanship of Francis Nonus Budd, younger brother of Dr William Budd, who had been Honorary Physician at the Infirmary (1847-1862) and who by then had a European reputation as an epidemiologist. The University College opened its doors in October 1876 located in two houses in Park

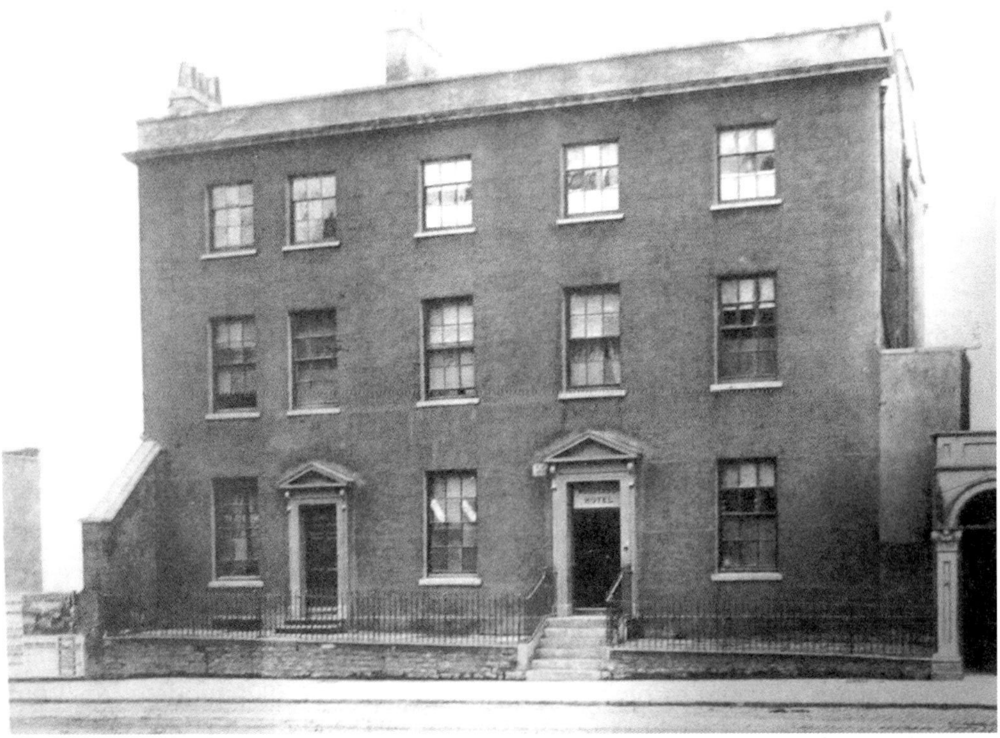

Figure 30. The University College's first premises in Park Row 1876.

Street. Students of the University College could either be registered or unregistered. If registered (costing one guinea) they could attend any lecture. Unregistered students paid 7 shillings per session.

The following year the College became affiliated to the Bristol Medical School which subscribed £1000 to the College. Thereafter the School nominated a member of the College Council each year. Robert William Tibbits MB MRCS was the first such appointee. He had been appointed as surgeon to the Infirmary in 1868 at the age of 26 years and during the next 10 years until his early death in 1878 was an active reformer. He may well have been responsible for inclusion of dental teaching in the College since he was the first lecturer in dental surgery. The entrance fee for the course in medicine was 5 guineas plus a further guinea for the use of the library at the Infirmary which claimed to have 2700 books. For clinical experience one became the pupil of a surgeon costing 12 guineas a year or 25 guineas for three years.

While there was no dental course at this time (it did not appear in the College Calendar until 1893/4) there is a brief section in the College Calendar of 1877/8 as follows:

DENTAL INSTRUCTION.

Classes will be formed for Dental Students in conformity with the regulations of the Royal College of Surgeons, provided a sufficient number of pupils present themselves.

Subjects.	Lecturers.	Fees. One course. £	s.	d.	Two courses. £	s.	d.
Dental Anatomy and Physiology	Mr. Atchley and Dr. Smith.	4	4	0	6	6	0
Dental Surgery	Mr. Coe & Mr. Tibbits	4	4	0	6	6	0
Dental Mechanics	Mr. T. C. Parson.	3	3	0	5	5	0
Dental Metallurgy	Mr. Coomber.	3	3	0			

Figure 31. Dental classes offered by the University College 1878 before there was a dental course. From the University College Calendar 1877/8 by kind permission of the University of Bristol Special Collections.

As well as these subjects the student of dentistry would also share lectures in physics, chemistry and biology with science students, and those in anatomy and physiology with the medical students. In many cases such students were in any case undertaking the course in medicine.

For clinical experience the student chose to attend either the Royal Infirmary or the General Hospital, on the days when the dental surgeons were present. (This freedom to choose continued until the Dental Hospital had opened in 1940). Mr. Cooke Parsons attended the General Hospital on two sessions each week. Parsons was originally a Bristol student, who took his medical degree in 1863. Quite what dental training he had, is not known but one must assume that he must have been a pupil at a dental practice in the city at some time. He retained his position as surgeon dentist at the General Hospital until 1890. The Bristol Infirmary had no dental surgeon so this training was provided by Mr. Tibbits until his death in 1878[30]. William Robert Ackland was then appointed as their first Dental Surgeon, attending the Infirmary on two sessions a week. The costs at this time are unknown but 10 years later the cost of becoming a pupil of the dental surgeon was 12 guineas for one year, 20 guineas for 2 years or 25 guineas for three years.

The year 1877 was a turning point for the dental profession. The clause in the Medical Act of 1858 allowed the Royal College of Surgeons to establish the Licentiate in Dental Surgery. In 1860 forty three candidates presented themselves for the first examination[31]. This established the division between qualified "dental surgeons" and unqualified "dentists". Both groups soon had their own representative associations and it was recognised that this could not continue. Samuel Cartwright found himself at the head of three such organisations and in due course chaired a national Dental Reform Committee to bring about dialogue between these groups. A full account of these negotiations may be read elsewhere[32].

By October 1877 the Royal College of Surgeons had agreed that all LDS candidates would have to pass a general examination before starting an LDS course. Thoughts of diploma examinations being held outside London began to be voiced. At a meeting in Manchester in May 1877 it was reported that a dental school was to be built in Dublin and that an appeal would be made to the Royal College of Surgeons in Ireland to establish their own LDS. A Dental Diploma Committee was then set up to coordinate these developments and meetings were held in Bristol, Leeds, Birmingham and Edinburgh all of which would have their own dental schools in due course. These deliberations produced changes in dental teaching at Bristol as elsewhere.

In July 1878 the first Dentists Act received the Royal Assent. From this time on no person would be allowed to call himself or herself "dentist" or "dental practitioner" unless they were registered with the General Medical Council. Those qualified to register (on payment of what was a large fee at the time of £5) were those holding the LDS of any medical authority and those then engaged in the practice of dentistry provided they applied before August 1879.

The early Dental Registers show that comparatively few who practised dentistry had gained a professional qualification. In the 1880s the words "in practice before 22 July 1878" were monotonously repeated against most names on every page of the book but the writing was on the wall for unqualified dental practice and changes at Bristol reflected this.

In the list of staff of the General Hospital contained in the Medical School calendar of 1878/9[33] the title "Lecturer on Dental Mechanics at the Medical School" appears for the first time under Cooke Parsons' name. However his name does not appear in the University College's list of 16 professors, lecturers and demonstrators and so one must assume this title had a different status. However unlike other dental lecturers listed at that time Parsons retained this teaching post for many years and so may be looked upon as the father of the Dental School with his lectureship regarded as the oldest dental teaching post in the infant University. In 1880/1 the General Hospital included for the first time Dental Surgery among its list of six "special departments".

Unfortunately relations between the University College and the surgeons of the two hospitals soon deteriorated. There was even a proposal by some members of the Infirmary medical staff that they should set up an rival medical school. Matters were resolved by the construction of a new College building on the newly acquired Tyndalls Park Estate which was occupied by the Medical School in 1880. Nothing of this building remains apart from the doorway in University Road bearing its Hippocratic aphorism translated by Chaucer as *"The life so short, the craft so long to learn"*.[34]

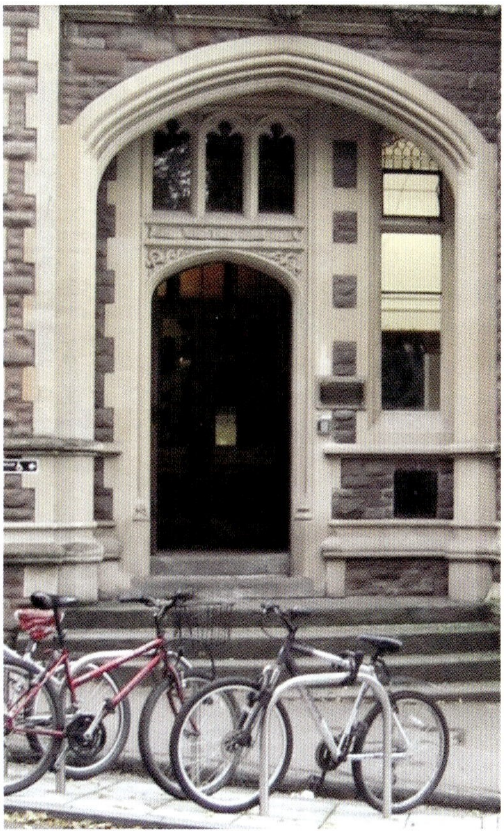

Figure 32. The only remaining evidence of the original Medical school

By 1888/9 the College's instructions to dental students included the statement that its lectures conformed to the requirements for the regulations of the Licentiate in Dental Surgery of the Royal College of Surgeons of England. It is no coincidence that in the same year the name of W. R. Ackland MRCS, LDSRCS, appeared as the first dental surgeon to the Infirmary. He now took over the post of Lecturer in Dental Mechanics from T. Cooke Parsons who became Lecturer in Dental Surgery.

By 1892 the College had built a medical wing, paid for by public subscription at a cost of nearly £8,000, on land in Tyndall's Park. (It is noteworthy that both Ackland and Parsons had contributed to the New Medical Wing Fund in 1891). Soon Bristol

University College dental students were travelling to the Royal College of Surgeons in either London, Glasgow or Dublin to take a qualifying examination. Robert Willcox was the first Bristol trained student to do so, taking the LDS FPS (Glasgow) in 1895. Three years later Frank Parlett was the first student of the College to take the LDSRCS (England). Robert Willcox was to become President of the Western Counties Branch of the BDA in 1913.

Thomas Cooke Parsons continued to hold his post as dental surgeon at the General Hospital until 1890. He left the University College two years later whereupon Ackland became Lecturer in Dental Surgery and a year later the Infirmary finally established a Department of Diseases of the Teeth. Ackland continued in this post for over thirty years, being succeeded in 1923 by Mr L E Claremont. The Lectureship in Dental Mechanics was taken over in 1893 for just a year by A W Hoffman after which, in 1894, C A Hayman was in charge of this subject until the end of the first World War. From 1894 to 1918 (twenty four years) the environment for the establishment of a dental school was nurtured by these two men. The one was from London the other a true Bristolian, for Hayman, like Parsons, had trained in Bristol. Hayman seems to have combined medicine with dentistry. He obtained his LDS in 1878 and took the MD at St Andrews in 1896 . In 1900 he was elected a Fellow of the Royal College of Surgeons of Ireland.

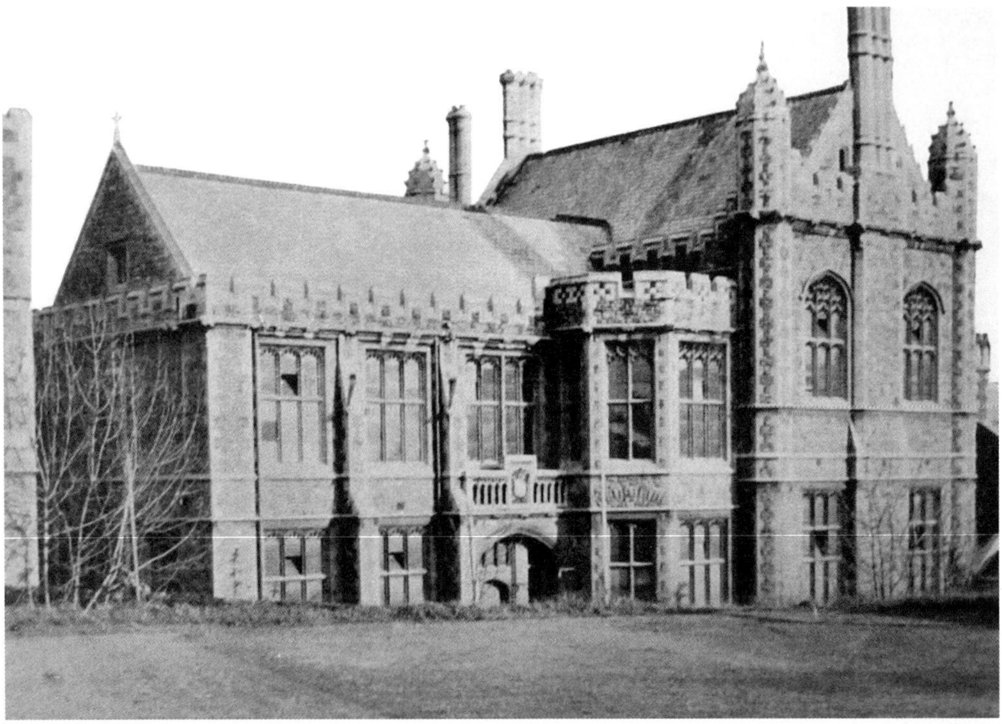

Figures 33. The new Medical School wing of 1892. From the University College Calendar by kind permission of the University of Bristol Special Collections.

When the medical wing was finished, the Medical School and the Bristol Medical School Library were incorporated within the College as its Faculty of Medicine and for the first time outline details of a dental course appear in the College Calendar as below.

DENTAL COURSES.

Dental Anatomy and Physiology.

This Course is given by the Professor of Physiology.

Dental Surgery.

Lecturer—W. R. ACKLAND, M.R.C.S., L.D.S., Dental Surgeon to the Bristol Royal Infirmary.

Dental Mechanics.

Lecturer—A. W. W. HOFFMAN, M.R.C.S., L.R.C.P., L.D.S.

Dental Metallurgy.

Lecturer—A. W. W. HOFFMAN, M.R.C.S., L.R.C.P., L.D.S.

Medical Tutor—W. M. STEVENS, M.D. Lond.

The Medical Tutor is in constant attendance, to assist Students in their studies.

Figure 34. Dental courses offered by the University College in 1892 From the University College Calendar 1892/3 with kind permission of the University of Bristol Special Collections.

Each course was £3-3s per year but there was a composite University College fee of £55 guineas for all instructions over the two year course.[35] At this time the Royal College of Surgeons of England required a candidate for the LDS to have received 2 years theoretical instruction, three years practical experience and to have attended a recognised hospital for at least two years practice of dental surgery.

The Professor of Physiology, under whose charge the course was run at this time, was G. Munro Smith who held this post from 1876 – 1899 when Professor A Stanley Kent took over. The same Munro Smith had been elected as a surgeon of the Royal Infirmary in 1897 and on his retirement in 1907 was to write the History of the Bristol Royal Infirmary published in 1917. He was highly influential in those years and was the only person to have his own room in the new medical wing and it was not until he left that this space became available for a laboratory of mechanical dentistry.

Students could attend the dental department of either the General Hospital or the Royal Infirmary for practical clinical instruction for which additional payment had to be made. It is clear that students, in theory at least , could attend both departments[36].

Mr. Cooke Parsons was at the General Hospital on Mondays and Thursday mornings, while Mr Ackland attended at the Infirmary at 1:00pm on Tuesdays and Fridays. What is not clear is how much supervision students received.

In 1896/7 the Dental Board of the United Kingdom, as the registration authority was now called, was beginning to make its presence felt and dental students were required to register with the General Medical Council for the first time. The two hospitals were also paying more attention to the needs of their students. By 1899 the Infirmary was claiming that there was a student room there "with lunches etc., available at moderate charges". Not to be outdone the General Hospital offered "a commodious room set apart for the use of all students with luncheons and teas supplied at moderate cost".

In 1901 the name of RM Hatch LDS appears for the first time as dental surgeon to the Bristol Infirmary for Sick Children and Women. The hospital which had opened its doors in 1866 moved to its present site on St Michaels Hill in 1885. It is not clear if Mr Hatch was involved in practical dental teaching but the fact that his session held at 11.00 am on Tuesday mornings did not clash with those of his other hospital dental colleagues might suggest that he was.

Moves to establish a University

Over the next few years the University College, its Faculty of Medicine and the dental course became better organised. From about the year 1906 the Faculty of Medicine began to demand more from the University College than the loose amalgamation of 1893. After much enquiry and discussion, comparing the financial provision for the Arts and Science Faculties, and also the cost to the medical student of training at Bristol and at other medical schools, a third and last stage was reached with the Faculty of Medicine's full integration with the College.

In April 1904 Charles Hayman became dental assistant to Mr Ackland and the following year two dental assistants were appointed, E. H. Lewis LDS and Frederick Perry LDS, and Dr. Leonard Moore became honorary dental anaesthetist. Munro Smith, a contemporary member of the consultant staff reported that

> *"The advantage of having a properly-equipped department, with expert dentists, and the many accessories necessary for tooth extraction, etc., was at once apparent, and the shrieks associated with this branch of surgery became confined to certain days."*[37]

In 1906 the University College Council passed the following resolution:

> *"The Dental Department be placed on a thoroughly satisfactory basis, with addition to the teaching staff and provision of laboratory accommodation to obviate a student having to become apprentice to some local practitioner".*

Space for this was made available in the ground floor of the medical wing later in that year. The Laboratory of Mechanical Dentistry has already been mentioned but there was now also a Dental Metallurgical Laboratory, which occupied space formerly taken up by a bookstore. In the same year the University College announced that successful negotiations with the Bristol General Hospital and Royal Infirmary meant that clinical instruction was now available to women " who are thus provided in Bristol with the means of full preparation for the medical profession".[38] Dentistry was quick to follow and Marjorie Jane White, who entered the school in 1910, qualified LDSRCS Eng in 1919. She was still practising in Bishopsgate London in 1954.

As new chemistry and physiology wings were being built for the Faculty of Medicine, the Physiology Laboratory in the Medical School was taken over and served as the Dental Department. Lectures in the College Calendar of 1906/7 are described for the first time as being held "in the Dental School".[39] There was a lecture timetable for the first time and recommended textbooks. In all the description of the dental course now had 8 pages devoted to it.

Despite appearing to have a more organised course the Dental School was still run in a haphazard way at this time. Some of the lectures were given at the lecturers' own homes because of the shortage of lecture rooms in the University College, and many were taken after 5 o'clock in the evening.[40] It is also interesting to see that the advice at this time was that if dental students could afford it they were "strongly advised to take the diploma of LRCP, MRCS". This view was not confined to Bristol. As late as 1940 those aspiring to a university dental career were advised to take a medical degree and it is notable that the "Bradlaw boys" who had taken this advice at Newcastle all ended up as Deans of Dental Schools, after the Second World War. This included Arthur Darling who would become the first Professor of Dental Surgery at Bristol (see Appendix 1).

The dental intake was still very small at the turn of the century. The Annual Reports of the College at this time mention the number of students studying for the various examinations leading to the LDS but not their names. However the records of Royal College of Surgeons supply the names of those who qualified as : 1903 F W Perry and W J Lennox; 1904 W E Boulter, A J Mundy and G H Smith; 1906 W J Jones and F C Nichols and in 1907 W H Ireland, C A Joll and C G Plumley.

By 1907 the University College boasted an Amalgamated Student Club into which the Medical Faculty's Football, Cricket and Rifle Clubs, the Medical Debating Society and Dramatic Society had all been merged. However the dental composition fees for the course had risen to 75 guineas. The total number of dental students in the College that year was six, George Fawn, being one of them. He was to qualify in 1912 and go on to play a major role in the future development of the School. It is perhaps no coincidence that a donation of 6 volumes had been made to the Medical Library in 1900 by James Fawn *and son*. James Fawn was a prominent bookseller of 42 Queens Road Bristol. He must have been a cultured man since he published a map of Bristol in 1890 and was a member of the Bristol and Gloucester Archaeological Society.

The pupilage system for dental mechanics was still in being. At the end of two years' pupilage the student spent the next six months making and fitting the six dentures and six crowns which then entitled him under G.M.C. regulations to be signed on to take the examination in mechanics. The impressions for these dentures and crowns were taken at the Bristol Royal Infirmary under the supervision of the honorary dental surgeon, but the mechanical work was completed in the workroom of the dental surgeon with whom the student was working.

The arrangements for clinical teaching at the Bristol Royal Infirmary at this time were far from satisfactory. The Dental Department originally had three rooms on the ground floor beneath the chapel the chairs were antiquated, and there was not even a full-time House Surgeon. The teaching was left entirely to three or four "honoraries".

The dental department in the General Hospital too had outgrown its accommodation and it was found necessary to take temporary accommodation in 3 and 4 Colston Parade which were fitted out as "waiting, extraction and operation rooms.[41] The

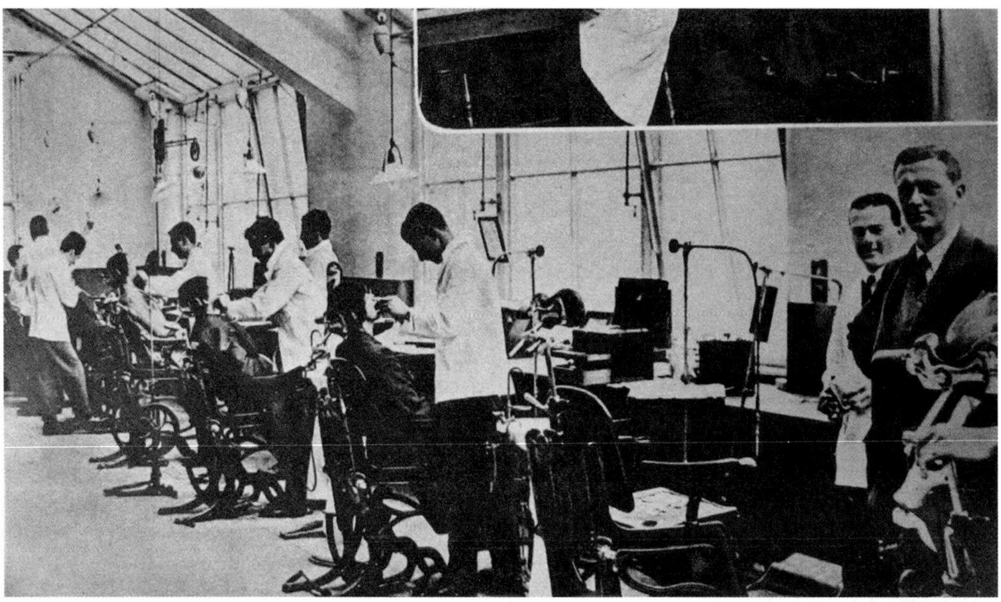

Figure 35. The rebuilt (1914) Dental Department of the General Hospital as it appeared in the University Appeal brochure of 1921 by kind permission of the University of Bristol Special Collections. The figure on the extreme right might be EA Dowling or LE Claremont.

problem was not fully resolved until a new dental department in the General Hospital itself was opened on July 27, 1914, a few days before war broke out. It occupied the ground floor of a new wing and consisted of a large room for conservative dentistry, a gas theatre with waiting and recovery rooms. Later an x-ray department and house surgeon's room were added. Mr. Dowling was appointed dental surgeon in the place of Mr. T.T. George who resigned in 1908, and Mr. Cottam was the house surgeon.

When the University of Bristol obtained its Royal Charter in 1909 the degrees of BDS and MDS and the LDS diploma were soon available. The University College Calendar of 1908-09 records the Officers in the Dental Department at this time as:

E A G Dowling, MRCS, LRCP, LDS, Lecturer in Dental Anatomy, Physiology and Dental Histology F W Perry, LDS, Demonstrator (in the same subjects)

Professor A F Stanley Kent, MA, FLS, FGS, Lecturer in Practical Physiology

Professor I Walker Hall, MD. Lecturer in Dental Bacteriology

Carey F Coombs. MD, MRCP, Demonstrator (in the same subject)

James F McBain, MA, Lecturer in Dental Metallurgy

W R Ackland, MRCS, LDS, Lecturer in Dental Surgery

C A Hayman, MD, FRCSI, LRCPI, LDS, Lecturer in Dental Mechanics

D C M Davis, BSc, FIC, Lecturer in Dental Materia Medica

In 1911 an external examiner in dental surgery was appointed. This was Charles Tomes MA, LDS, FRS, FRCS later to be knighted and the son of Sir John Tomes FRS. It was a wise choice for, since the death of his father in 1895, Charles had become the leading figure in the advance of the dental profession. He had been nominated by the Privy Council to a seat on the General Medical Council in 1898 and served on the 1917 Ackland Committee[42] whose proposals would lead to the passing of the 1921 Dentists Act which finally prohibited the practice of dentistry by unregistered persons. Tomes had taken the LDSRCS in 1869[43] and was now one of its examiners. He was on the staff at the Dental Hospital of London (later to become the Royal Dental Hospital) as well as being the author of the two standard dental texts. Just for good measure under the name of Charles Sissmore he painted in oils and watercolours, and at least once exhibited at the Royal Academy!

At Bristol CJ Kelsey and WJ Lennox were the first to achieve the new BDS degree in 1911, but quite what form this examination with Charles Tomes took is not clear. Kelsey had been qualified for 13 years, having achieved the LDSRPS Glasgow in 1898. (He would go on to achieve his MDS (UBrist) in 1914, the first Bristol student to do so, although Ackland as a member of staff had achieved this in 1912). Lennox on the other hand had been qualified for a mere 8 years. He had taken the LDSRCS England in 1903 at which examination he may well have met the same Charles Tomes. So one imagines that the examination for these two "students" on this occasion would have taken the form of a friendly discussion between professional colleagues! But why did they bother to take a dental degree when they had both already achieved a registerable dental qualification? As each went on to play an important role in the development of academic dentistry at Bristol it seems that they had realized that to have any influence in the University they would need to hold a degree. Lennox remained on the staff until 1941 and thus had a connection with the School for almost fifty years.

George Fawn who qualified BDS Bristol in 1912 was the first student to do so. Some time after the turn of the century he had been apprenticed to his mother's brother,

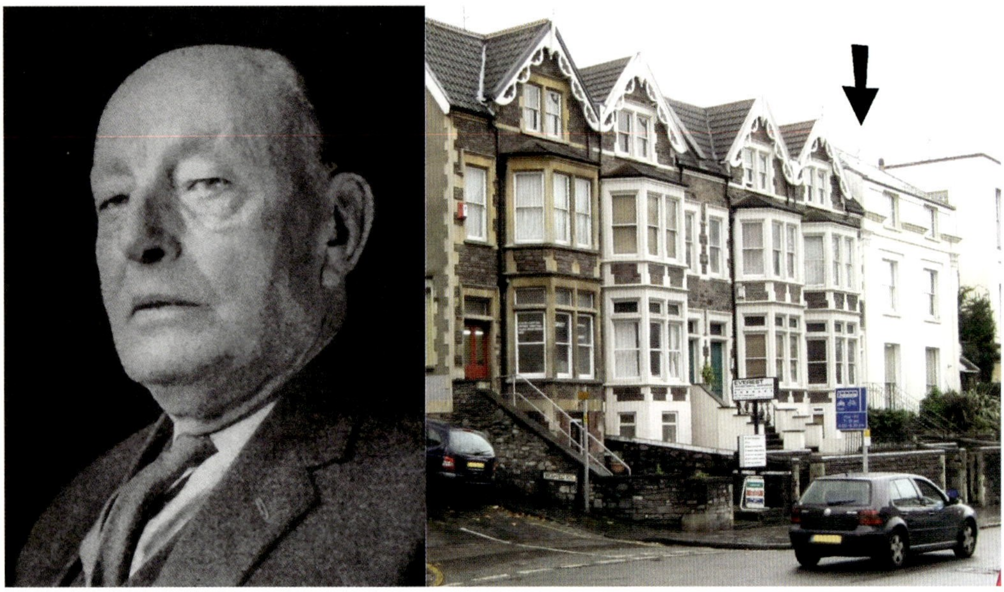

Figure 36a. Mr G Fawn MDS, FDS, MRCS, LRCP. 36b. The Hayman practice in Cheltenham Road, where he worked.

Frank Hayman. Frank practised at 197 Cheltenham Road[44]. Simultaneously with this pupilage George Fawn had undertaken the University College's medical and dental courses. From time to time Frank Hayman used to stand in for W. R. Ackland at the Infirmary.

Clinical conditions and supervision in the Royal Infirmary were still very poor at this time. In 1910 because nothing had been done to address their grievances the students approached Mr. Dowling, who had been appointed lecturer in 1907. He invited them to attend the Bristol General Hospital department for their clinical work where he also held the appointment of dental surgeon. All but two accepted his invitation to the obvious consternation of the Infirmary. It is possible that George was one of the two who decided to remain at the Infirmary. (He was living at 27 Claremont Road, Bristol 7 in 1911 which would have been walking distance from the University and Infirmary and also very convenient for his uncle's practice in the Cheltenham Road. The longer journey to the General Hospital would have been more difficult).

Almost immediately the University decided to contribute half the salary (£50), for a dental house surgeon post at the Bristol Infirmary to ensure that constant supervision of students could be provided. The following year George took and gained the LRCP London, the MRCS Eng, and the BDS Bristol and was appointed to this new post. Curiously Fawn's name first appears on the Medical Register with an entry dated 26th July 1912 but on the Dentists Register not until 4th June 1913. However there was no need for dentists to register at this time and perhaps it was only after he gained a dental appointment at the Infirmary that he felt this to be a prudent move.

George Fawn and Frederick C Nichols served with the Royal Army Medical Corps in the First World War and both had achieved the rank of Captain. Nichols, who was attached to the 4th Battalion the Staffordshire Regiment, was awarded the Military Cross. He had entered University College as a student in 1902 and qualified both medically and dentally (LDSRCS) in 1906. In 1909 he succeeded Charles Hayman as Assistant Dental Surgeon to the Bristol Royal Infirmary, and in 1922 succeeded Ackland as its Dental Surgeon, a post which he held until his untimely death in 1940. This was a serious loss for the staff of the new school in Lower Maudlin Street, which was felt by all his colleagues. For many years Nichols had also been the Lecturer in Dental Anatomy and according to Stoy (1947) many recalled with mixed feelings his rather cryptic discussions on the morphology of the teeth. Like Parsons, Hayman, Ackland and Dowling, who had preceded him as Lecturer in Dental Anatomy, Nichols was a craftsman and set a high standard of conservative dentistry for the students to emulate.

The University College at Bristol had been the first in the country to admit women on the same basis as men*. However, women were forbidden to take examinations in medicine until 1906. Of the few women students at Bristol University in its early years Marjorie Jane White was the first to gain a dental qualification - the LDSRCS (England) in 1915. The first LDS (Bristol) was awarded to Violette Bourgeois in 1919 but the first BDS (Bristol) degree was not gained by a woman until Muriel Emma Strode Cosh achieved this in 1930.

Up until the First World War the pupilage system for dental mechanics was still in being and it was not necessary to attend the dental department of a hospital in order to acquire the necessary clinical experience. Many pupils were used as cheap

---

* Several interesting accounts of these times are contained in Jerrard J. Reminiscences. University of Bristol Womens Club. Bristol,1997.

labour and received little instruction. Preferred alternatives had been suggested as long ago as 1891[45] but this less expensive route did not require the student to have the qualifications for University entrance yet still prepared them to take the LDS and become registered dentists. Professor Edward Fawcett FRS, an anatomist and the Dean of the Faculty of Medicine at Bristol (1909-1934), seems to have taken a particular interest in improving dental education generally and in Bristol in particular. He attended an early meeting of the Association of Dental Teachers of the North, held in Manchester in about 1917 and made the proposal that private pupilage should be abolished which was carried unanimously. The result was that the Dental Mechanical Laboratory at Bristol came into line with the Physiological and other laboratories and the students paid an annual fee. By this time a Dentists Act Committee had been set up of which more will be said later.

The dental course was slowly becoming an important part of the Faculty's activity. Sadly the earliest Medical Board minutes of the University have been lost but it is clear from the first available (handwritten) minutes dated May 19th 1911 that there was already a Dental Subcommittee by this time, which was chaired by Ackland. It reported to the Board of Faculty on which he also served. By the beginning of the session 1913/14 it was being reported that:

> "There were 37 dental students in the Faculty. Of these 5 were working for the BDS of the University of Bristol, 3 for the LDS of the same University and 29 for the LDS of the conjoint Board."
>
> "The great proportion of dental students to the whole number of students in the Faculty is very significant and invites very careful consideration. The numbers are rapidly growing , and it will be seen from a later table that there actually entered last October 12 dental students as against 15 medical students. I venture to express the opinion that we ought to have a first class dental school, and that it is in this direction that the Faculty of Medicine is likely to grow. The dental mechanical laboratory has been a great success, 10 students having worked in it during the past year .Should more come it will be necessary to increase the accommodation therein. To make it of still greater utility to the students we shall require to have more instruction provided in it and more opportunity that at present holds for "gold" work."[46]

Numbers attending classes were still very small in that years ranging from 7 in Operative Dental Surgery to only 3 in Materia Medica.

The Bristol MDS had been established when the University was founded but there was no provision for this, or the BDS degree to be award with honours. Then in May 1914 C.J. Kelsey submitted his dissertation "Oral bacteria exhibiting streptobacillary characters" for the Bristol MDS. At the next meeting of the Board a proposal was made to allow both degrees to be awarded with honours. At the following Board meeting it was announced that Senate had approved this new regulation and at the same Board meeting Kelsey was awarded his MDS with honours![47]

Despite the fact that numbers at Bristol were thought to be growing, the GMC circulated all dental schools in April 1915 expressing its concern at the shortage of qualified dentists. It was pointed out that the number of registered qualified dentists had increased by little more than 100 since the passing of the 1878 Dentists Act. In view of this the GMC asked whether the answer was to lower the entrance requirements.[48] Ackland's reply gives an alternative explanation.

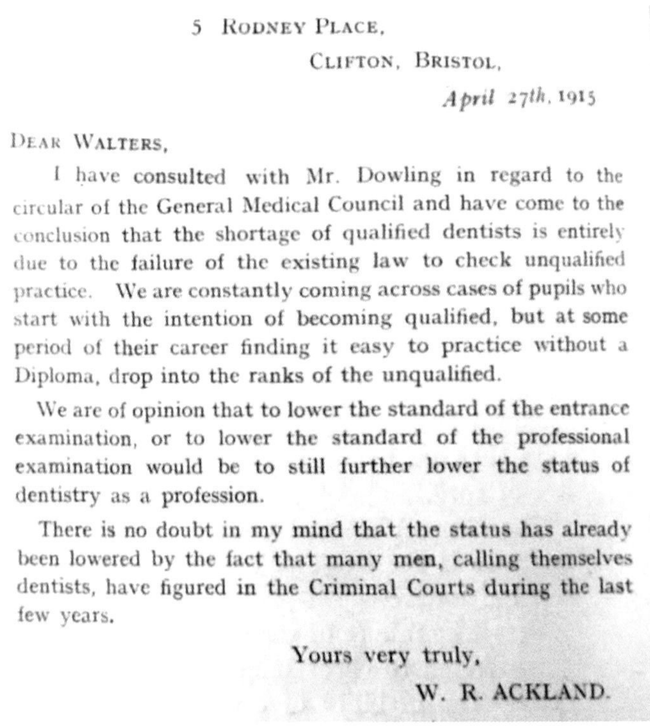

5 Rodney Place,
Clifton, Bristol,
April 27th, 1915

Dear Walters,

I have consulted with Mr. Dowling in regard to the circular of the General Medical Council and have come to the conclusion that the shortage of qualified dentists is entirely due to the failure of the existing law to check unqualified practice. We are constantly coming across cases of pupils who start with the intention of becoming qualified, but at some period of their career finding it easy to practice without a Diploma, drop into the ranks of the unqualified.

We are of opinion that to lower the standard of the entrance examination, or to lower the standard of the professional examination would be to still further lower the status of dentistry as a profession.

There is no doubt in my mind that the status has already been lowered by the fact that many men, calling themselves dentists, have figured in the Criminal Courts during the last few years.

Yours very truly,
W. R. Ackland.

Figure 37. The Bristol reply to the GMC letter of April 1915. From the Medical Faculty Board Minutes with kind permission of the University of Bristol Special Collections.

With the onset of the Great War, the number of dental students rapidly declined as many volunteered for the Forces. During the years of 1914-18, the School carried on under great difficulties. By 1916, the number enrolled on the Dental Mechanics course had dropped to one – Edward James Tucker – who was the first to take the Bristol LDS in 1920. Up until that time it was customary to take the LDS of either Glasgow or the London Royal Colleges.

When in 1919 men came back from the First World War there was an influx of 50 new students. The pressure was first felt in the Medical School's dental laboratory which had to be enlarged to accommodate fifty students. On one occasion twenty-five sat for the same examination, and the total number of students in the dental school was now 100. At the Bristol Royal Infirmary the new Edward VII building, which had been occupied by the military during the war, was returned to civilian use and the conservation room, extraction rooms, etc, were then transferred to its first floor - an arrangement which lasted for only a few years. The department was soon moved again, this time to the garden of the old building near the Cottage where it remained until the opening of the present Dental Hospital on the opposite side of Lower Maudlin Street thirty years later.

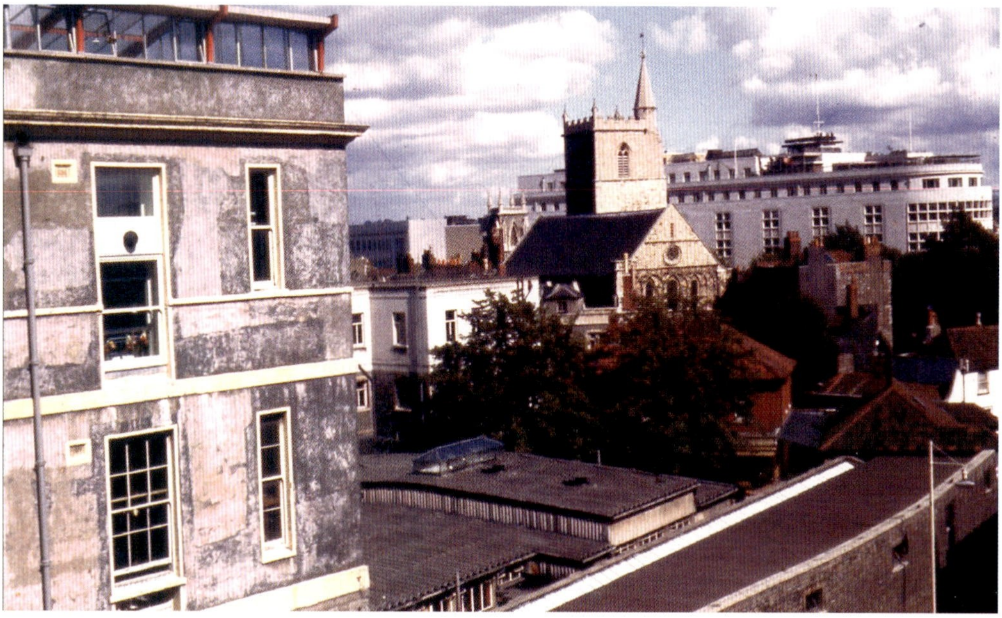

Figure 38. Showing the Old Royal Infirmary "garden" today .The roof of what had been the BRI dental department before 1940 is visible in the bottom right corner.

In the late 1920s some trades unions and "approved societies" had introduced a dental benefit as part of their health insurance schemes. In the next few years some fifty contributory schemes were formed in Bristol and the Corporation of Bristol also sent "necessitous persons" for treatment[49]. The accommodation of the two hospital departments became inadequate for the large post-war influx of students and their patients. By 1922 the position had become acute. According to Stoy [34] the Dental Students' Society minutes contain many references to the students' strong feelings on the subject:

> "October 6th 1922: *Mr Simkiss asked if anything specific had been done in the matter of lack of Dental Chairs at the Bristol Royal Infirmary. Mr R C Price, speaking for the Committee formed to deal with this matter, answered in the negative".*

At a meeting held three weeks later, the Society asked for a conference to be arranged between the University Authorities, the Working Committee of the Bristol Royal Infirmary and the dental students, to discuss the insufficient number of dental chairs provided at the Bristol Royal Infirmary.

It was reported that:

> *"Not only were students being deprived of sufficient chairside work, but the patients suffered in that they were kept waiting for an hour or more or were sent away and asked to attend at a later date - which did not encourage future visits."*

The Committee were asked:-

> *"to endeavour to arrange further supervision of conservative work by the Honorary Dental Surgeons - especially in the mornings".*

The minutes of the Board of Faculty indicate that either the University did not feel this was their problem or else it wished to conceal it from the Senate for there is no mention of this, apart from an entry in the minutes of 28th April 1922 proposing that:

> *"In order to meet the convenience of certain final Dental Students who are on grant, it recommends that a supplementary final examination be held for the LDS in October 1922. It makes this recommendation because, owing to circumstances over which the students have no control they have not been able to give as much time to the work as they would have done under ordinary conditions."*

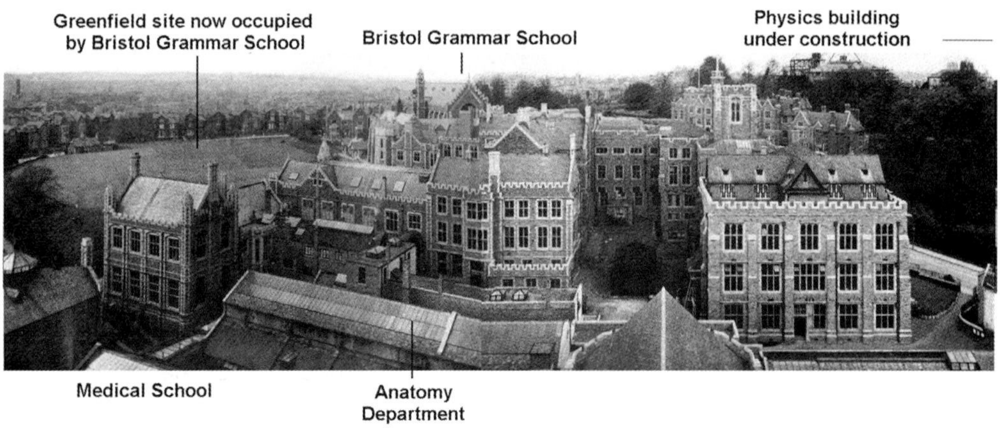

Figure 39. A composite view formed from two 1925 photographs showing the Medical School in 1925 .The Dental Laboratory was later located in the old Anatomy Department , see Figure 41.

Many of such difficulties were the result of a long term rivalry between the Bristol General Hospital and Bristol Royal Infirmary. In 1919 Sir George Newman had undertaken a survey of UK medical schools on behalf of the Government and had commented that Bristol was "at sixes and sevens". Sir George Wills attempted to break the deadlock at Bristol by offering to build a new hospital on the Downs if the two hospitals could resolve their differences. The Minutes of the Faculty Board of 12th June 1919 speak confidently that this would be accomplished in a few years. Sadly the two parties could not agree and the site is now occupied by St Monica's Home of Rest.

The same year saw an approach to the Faculty from the Acting Medical Officer of Health for Bristol who was intending to open a school dental clinic in Portland Square. He suggested collaboration in the appointment of a dental surgeon.[50] A more radical proposal was to be made two years later made by the County Medical Officer for Health and School Medical Officer for Gloucester. At this time unqualified dental dressers were used in schools' clinics to undertake work under supervision. In view of this the proposal was made that Bristol dental students should attend his clinics as dressers to gain experience. A two month period for final year students was agreed in November 1920. There was the proviso that the supervising School Dental Officer should be appropriately qualified so that they could be appointed as Recognised Teachers.[51] So began what is now almost a century of cooperation between University and Community Dental Service in neighbouring counties. The practice of employing dressers was not finally abolished until 1925.

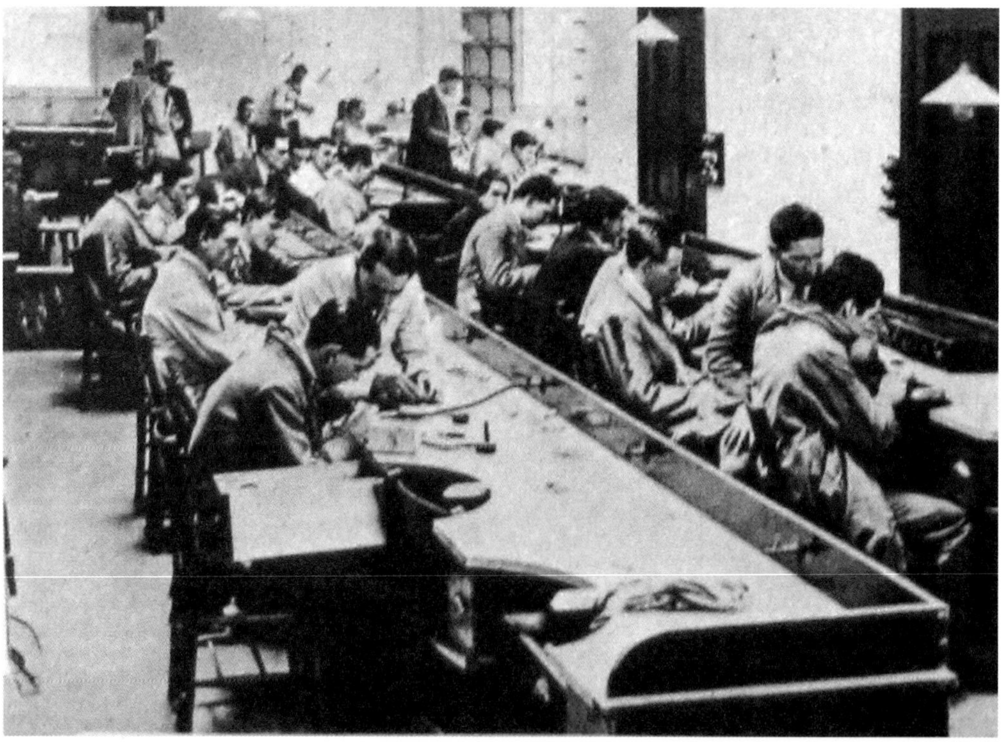

Figure 40. The Medical School's Dental Laboratory in 1921. It had been recently enlarged to accommodate 50 students From the University Appeal brochure of 1921. (By kind permission of the University of Bristol Special Collections)

There had been an earlier request to the Board this time from Mr CJ Kelsey as chairman of the Local Advisory Technical Committee. This was to allow the dental laboratory to be put at the disposal of disabled soldiers so they could train as dental mechanics. This was readily agreed and proved to be very successful.[52] It is the first time that a technical training course is mentioned in the University's Medical Board Minutes.

At the end of 1920 the GMC finally agreed that it was no longer necessary for dental students to attend the full course of lectures on medicine and surgery provided for medical students. The presented the University with a problem. Who then was to provide lectures thought appropriate for the dental course? The answer was to seek applications for clinical lectureships from the registrars in medicine and surgery who would be paid a small honorarium.[53]

Chapter 5

THE DENTAL HOSPITAL AND SCHOOL 1921-1945

By the end of the First World War the pressure to establish a national register of appropriately qualified dentists was irresistible. In 1917 Sir Francis Dyke Acland had been appointed Chairman of an interdepartmental Committee "to inquire into the extent and gravity of the evils of dental practice by persons not qualified under the Dentists Act [1878].". Based on its recommendations a bill was introduced into parliament which eventually became the Dentists Act of 1921. The Act established the Dental Board of the United Kingdom and Acland was appointed its first Chairman - a position he held until his death. The Board's recommendations were considered, and in general ratified, by the General Medical Council. Registration as a dentist now required the payment of an annual fee of £5, a great deal of money in those days, but this was put to good use by the Board's 13 far sighted members. During the time of its existence (1921-1956) the Board disbursed £500,000 in supporting dental education by giving grants to dental schools and bursaries to hundreds of dental students. It also did a great deal to raise professional standards through lectures and publications.

In November 1920 Norman King of the GMC wrote to all those Universities which offered dental courses asking if they would run special courses and examinations for those who held no dental qualification.[54] This and a similar approach by "The National Dental Association"[55] received the response from the Faculty's Dental Board at Bristol that the most appropriate course of study was that for the LDS UBrist! Shortly before this its chairman WR Ackland had been appointed to the Panel of Examiners for the Dental Board of the United Kingdom so one imagines the response was the party line from the new Board.

In 1922 EA Dowling resigned his post and the vacant lectureship in operative dental surgery was filled by LE Claremont.[56] A year later year Ackland retired and after some deliberation by its dental sub committee the Medical Board agreed that dental surgery and operative dental surgery should be taught together and Claremont was now given both responsibilities.

The following year a further letter was received from the Dental Board of the GMC this time asking if the University would be prepared to institute post registration lectures in dental surgery.[57] As these were to be for registered dentists and not a back door means to qualification the Faculty agreed. It would seem that this was the beginning of the concept of "lifelong learning" for dentists. In 1924 the same Dental Board inspected the University's LDS course which was found to be "sufficient", a term which is still used today. The year also saw the appearance of the term " Dental Tutors" used by the Faculty at Bristol for those hospital staff who undertook teaching. One early such appointee was EK Tratman, later Professor Tratman, of whom more will be said later.[58]

In 1925 the number of LDS diplomas awarded was 27, the peak following the post war bulge, with 14 more given in the following year. The following year 11 students qualified LDS but only one with BDS. In fact only 7 BDS degrees were awarded by Bristol between 1911 and 1930!

Another first was the agreement by the University in 1928 to run postgraduate courses for Royal Naval dental officers,[59] but the proposal by the BDA for an additional dental qualification to be established in "Public Dentistry" seems to have fallen on stony ground.[60] Another far sighted proposal was that radiology should be taught to dental students but this too seems to have got no further.[61]

Dental education now moved rapidly moved out of an era which had been dominated by apprenticeships into one of full time study in University dental schools. In October 1929 Claremont resigned his Bristol lectureship to take up the directorship of the Eastman Dental Clinic in London which was opened on 20 November 1931 by the American Ambassador in the presence of the Prime Minister Neville Chamberlain. This was to become the first postgraduate school in the UK. In the same month congratulations were being offered by the Bristol Faculty Board to Tratman who had been appointed Professor of Dental Surgery in Singapore.[62]

Professor R J Brocklehurst, who was appointed to the Chair of Physiology in 1930 and was a member of the Dental Hospital Management Committee from 1940, contributed the following information to Dr. Hugh Levers in 1963.[63]

> *"In 1928 the University applied to the Board for a grant to cover the cost of an addition to the Dental Mechanics Laboratory, then on the main University site. The Board's Treasurers visited Bristol that year and expressed dissatisfaction with the clinical facilities in the Bristol Royal Infirmary's and the Bristol General Hospital's Dental Departments. The Board refused to consider a grant to the University before the latter had gone into the question of (establishing) a single Dental School."*

In 1929 the UK Dental Board's Treasurers again visited Bristol to look at sites suggested by the University for a new Dental School. These were:

(1) in the grounds of the General Hospital;

(2) in the grounds of the Infirmary;

(3) at Canynge Hall, then a hall of residence.

The Treasurers favoured (2) and in 1930 the Dental Board resolved to make a grant of £5,000 towards the cost of a new Dental School and Hospital on this site. In spite of the Board's recommendation the University prepared plans for the conversion of Canynge Hall, on the grounds that the University could not expect to have freedom of action in a building which was not the absolute property of the University. One of the GMC treasurers again came to Bristol and expressed his disapproval of the Canynge Hall site, chiefly due to its remote situation.

Matters were precipitated when the Dental Board of the UK reported unsatisfactorily on the teaching arrangements in Bristol and it was under this pressure that the University Council in 1931 gave priority to the building of a Dental Hospital. Even so nine years were to elapse before the Hospital was opened, as a site had still to be agreed. Similar delays were to occur in the appointment of the first full time lecturer in orthodontics which was recommended and approved by the Medical Board in 1935.[64] However inexplicably it was to take another 30 years until Mr Derek Seel was appointed to that post!

In 1935 the University's eyes fell on 15-18 Lower Maudlin Street –including the shop of Messrs. Cole and Pottow. A member of the UK Dental Board came to see the site and expressed approval; the offer of the grant appears then to have been renewed on condition that the University established a school for all dental teaching in premises belonging to them. Thus in 1936, the University purchased the site at a cost of £6,000 and other adjacent properties for £1,625 and £8,000.

It was about this time that, during the annual conference of the British Dental Association, it was resolved to form a committee to exchange views on matters affecting dental education. An inaugural meeting of what was to become the Dental Education Advisory Council took place at the Royal Dental Hospital London on January 31st 1931. Bristol Dental Hospital was represented by Professor E Fawcett FRS the long standing Dean of Medicine.[65] The new advisory council; was to play a key role in providing an authoritative consensus to the General Medical Council on educational standards in dentistry. It is perhaps of note that Fawcett was the only Professor at the meeting, all other representatives being practising dentists holding dental teaching appointments.

In 1937 the University reported that the city authorities required the Lower Maudlin Street frontage to be set back. Fortunately the University had been able to purchase a neighbouring site, which would compensate for the loss of accommodation resulting from the City's requirements. This was perhaps the old brass foundry built on the site of the Penitentiary (See Chapter 1) The Architect, Mr Eustace Button, was appointed in 1936 and the first estimates were approved by the University in 1937, subject to the approval of the Dental Board. A member of the Board again visited Bristol and expressed the opinion that the building as planned on the Lower Maudlin Street site would accommodate the proposed number of students with room for later expansion.

The University accepted the Board's £5,000 grant towards the new school building and later a further grant of £1500 towards the cost of chairs and dental units. The School built by Messrs. H Willcock & Co was formally opened on April 10, 1940 by Dr Stanley H Badock, Pro-Chancellor of the University and Mr E L Sheridan, Chairman of the Dental Board. The total cost was £83,000.

While the new Dental Hospital opened officially on April 10th 1940 it had been open to clinical students in January. The new premises were a revelation to clinical students who had until that time had experienced the old BRI dental department on the opposite side of Maudlin Street (see Hugh Leech's account below).

The meeting of the Dental Management Committee of the 29th of January 1940 confirmed the following among the regulations for the new Hospital:

1. The institution shall be known as the University of Bristol Dental Hospital (*note that the addition of "and School" to the title came many years later*).
2. The object of the institution shall be to afford treatment in all cases of disease and injury of the teeth and associated parts to persons suitable for treatment at a hospital; also the provision of artificial teeth and dental appliances to such people.
4. The hospital shall be managed by the Council of the University through the Committee of Management.
5. The Management Committee shall have power to appoint a House Committee.
21. The Hospital shall be the Dental School of the University of Bristol.

From January 1940 no dental out-patients were treated at the Infirmary or General Hospital. This decision had been facilitated by the earlier amalgamation between BRI and BGH which became effective on September 15th, 1939. The Dental Board of the GMC at this time thought that the new clinical and teaching facilities would be sufficient to accommodate 25 students each year. This brought to an end a situation in which neither University laboratories nor hospital departments had been adequate and in which students had to be continually on the move between lecture room, laboratory and hospital to accomplish their studies.

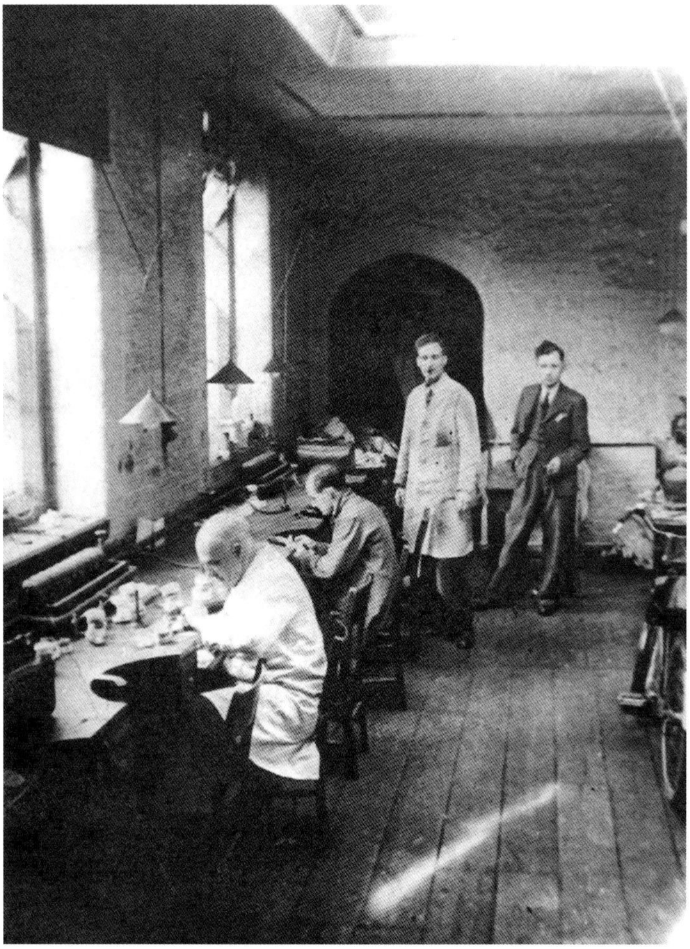

Figure 41. The dental laboratory in 1930.

The original dental laboratory which had taken over space in the old Anatomy Department was still in use until the opening of the Dental Hospital in Lower Maudlin Street .This is shown above as it was in the 1930s. In the foreground is the late Mr Dennis, standing in the white coat is the much loved Mr. Sidney Mattock who finally retired as chief technician in 1978. The Gladstone bag on the end of the bench was used to take "bites" ,"try-ins" etc to the dental departments of the General Hospital and Royal Infirmary using the laboratory's bicycle just visible in the right on the picture.

Mr Mattock who ran the laboratory, was noted for his pipe which never left his mouth. Ivor Robinson joined this lab just before the war as the youthful apprentice and he too rose to become Chief Technician and Chief Dental Instructor in the School. Another character at this time was Henry Davis, a heavy smoker. Immediately after WW II all ex service students and technicians smoked. Henry, supplemented his own supply from packets left unwisely by students in the pockets of their lab coats.[66]

The new Hospital and School

The new Dental Hospital was governed by the Dental Management Committee which was responsible to the University Council . It consisted initially of:

The Chairman of the University Council.

Treasurer of the University.

The Vice Chancellor.

The Dean of the Faculty of Medicine.

Four other members appointed by the University Council.

The Dental Assistant Dean (Mr P Stoy).

Two representatives of the Honorary Dental Staff (George Fawn and Mr Kettlewell).

Two representatives of the Bristol Royal Hospital.

Chairman of the City Health Committee.

The Medical Officer of Health of the City.

The first meeting of this group appears to have been held on 4th December 1939 and the subsequent minutes record the efforts made during late 1939 and the early moths of 1940 to equip and staff the new building. In fact most of this work was carried out by George Fawn, Mr Kettlewell and especially PJ Stoy who in January 1940 had been made Dental Assistant Dean to the Dean of the Faculty of Medicine.[67] He it was who chaired the Dental House Committee which was responsible for the day to day running of the School.[68]

The School soon had eight clinical lecturers and three assistants, a sister (Miss MG Thomson) with a staff nurse, and an almoner/secretary. There were 7 honorary dental surgeons who each received an £40 per annum. There was an SHO paid £150 p.a. and two junior dental house surgeons each paid £100 p.a.[69]

The expenditure for the Hospital for its first complete year of 1940/1 was £4404 Hospital income was from "dentures" (£2000) "non dentures" (£1000) and the Hospital Contributory Scheme. This left a deficit of £1154 in that year. The School's expenditure was £3100. Its income was derived from student fees of £2600 and a £600 grant from the Dental Board of the General Medical Council.

Hugh Leech BDS LDS (UBrist 1944) was one of the first intake of students to the new building. He was to become a distinguished consultant orthodontist who was in turn Secretary and then President of British Society for the Study of Orthodontics. He provides a vivid account of his time as an undergraduate at Bristol during the Second World War based on his diaries of those years. It is a curious fact that while Hugh was fire-watching on the roof of the newly opened Bristol Dental School, Arthur Darling, who was soon to become the University's first dental professor was learning anatomy for his 2nd MB from (later Professor) Howard Tonge as they fire watched on the roof of the Durham Medical School.

From the diaries of Hugh Leech

1939

On 2nd October 1939 I registered as an undergraduate student at the Wills Memorial University tower in Clifton. My immediate purchases were a second-hand gown for ten shillings and a microscope for £2 10s 0d. I enrolled in the Mortimer House Men's Hall of Residence near the Clifton Suspension bridge (Mortimer House, Mortimer Street now a Nursing Home) and at first shared a second floor study-bedroom with a fellow dental student, as extra accommodation in the building was required for the recently evacuated students from Kings College, London; their refuge from the anticipated air-raids on the capital following the outbreak of hostilities. Little did they then realise that such events would not escape them!

There were about forty-five students in residence and my first impressions were favourable, in spite of the attendance at dinner that first evening (wearing the obligatory gown). A shadow was cast by the long and dreary "welcoming" speech by the Warden, Mr "Bags" Turner, which was full of what we considered to be petty restrictions. Some of these, however, were necessary because of the possible results of enemy action and the strict observance of the "black-out" and air-'raid precautions, including the correct use of hose-pipes, sand-buckets and stirrup-pumps. These were needed for the extinction of fires from incendiary bombs and any unnecessary tampering with them was a "sending-down" offence.

Before retiring we were escorted to the basement air-raid shelter and,' instructed in the correct procedures to be followed on the sounding of the air-raid siren. Formal lectures started the next morning in the main buildings in University Road and as far as I was concerned, consisted of the 1st B.D.S. pre-clinical course. The first was in the theory of chemistry by Dr Rixon, starting at 9.00 a.m. Whilst more formal dress and gown were required by the lecturers, students were allowed a certain degree of sartorial licence, men wearing a blazer or sports jacket with flannel trousers and sporting their recently acquired faculty tie, whilst the women usually wore the traditional skirt and jumper. Nylon had not yet been invented, so during the very cold winter to come they were obliged to wear the less attractive knee-length woollen stockings. Some students made up for this much later, when the availability of nylon stockings materialised with the advent of American service personnel! After the one hour chemistry lecture we moved immediately to the Biology Department for another hour's lecture in this subject by Major Jock Sloan, who was also the Commandant of the University Senior Training Corps.

After only a short break we strolled up to the Royal Fort for the final lecture in Physics by Dr Piper. By this time our minds and bodies were showing signs of fatigue and as this final lecture theatre was relatively palatially furnished with "plush" seats, it took some effort to remain awake and attentive in spite of the riveting presentation of the subject.

Practical laboratory work took place in the afternoons, the most memorable being that of Dr OCM Davies in chemistry. He was usually known as "Beak" - an elderly gentleman with degrees in both medicine and law. He treated "his boys and girls" as he called us with a slightly patronising attitude. As we now regarded ourselves as very much "grown up" this rankled a little at first, but soon subsided when we appreciated his very fine teaching.

On 24th October I formally became a student of the University by attending the Matriculation Ceremony and shaking hands with the Vice Chancellor, Sir Thomas Loveday, followed by the signing of the University Roll. Our Chancellor, of course, was Winston Churchill, who had yet to become Prime Minister and head of the coalition government for the remainder of the War. Fortunately there was an abundance of facilities for relaxation and those at the university union building - the imposing Victoria Rooms - were soon put to very good use. The Freshers Social Dance early in the term was a great success; quite informal and a splendid opportunity to meet members of the other faculties and the King's College guests.

Apart from its large hall and stage, where many notable performances were to take place, it housed the refectory run by a very pleasant and efficient manageress in the form of Mrs. Underdown. The gymnasium and bars were to occupy many of my happy hours, in spite of the fact that the men's bar was out of bounds to the students of the fair sex! The barman was an ex. Royal Navy boxing champion, Frank Treasure who, with his wife, were devoted to the welfare of their clientele, especially when they over-indulged!

The magnificent sports grounds at Coombe Dingle and the new Squash and Fives Courts in Woodland Road completed the picture and I was fortunate enough to become a member of the University 1st soccer XI this term.

This first term then proved to be most enjoyable and free from any enemy activity; in fact it was difficult to believe that the Country was at war and the period was generally described as "the phoney war".

We were kept very busy with our studies and end of term exams also extra-mural activities, but the latter rarely involved fraternising with the opposite sex. Believe it or not, we were all far more concerned with ensuring a good academic achievement for our examiners at this stage of our careers.

One incidence of light relief occurred towards the end of term when the residents of Mortimer House regaled themselves in female attire and make-up prior to attending a debate at Clifton Hill House women's hall of residence. The motion "That cosmetics are a necessity" was carried almost unanimously, thanks to our support. A good time was had by all especially as this was one of the few occasions when men and women students were allowed to socialize officially!

However, on returning home to Mortimer House we were confronted by a considerable number of envious inmates from our rival establishment Wills Hall. A general boisterous fracas ensued which was far from appreciated by either the Warden of Mortimer or the very apprehensive lay air-raid warden in his tin-hat and authoritative arm-band, who kept blowing his whistle and threatening us with arrest as so-called "rioters". The air-raid siren had already sounded and he obviously was not too sure whether we were indeed students or disguised enemy paratroopers.

The following day we were paraded before our own Warden to be censured and warned that any recurrence of our outrageous behaviour would result not only in being dismissed from Mortimer, but even sent down. Needless to say, a subsequent request for lady guests to be allowed an invitation to Sunday tea was firmly denied.

The University Rag Week in December was not forbidden by war-time restrictions and proved to be very successful. Our barrel-organ and collecting box excursion to most of the City centre resulted in a considerable donation to the Salvation Army War Work Appeal. I went down for the Christmas vacation with a feeling of considerable satisfaction having matured from my school-days to manhood! Little did I realise then that the real maturity was destined to manifest itself in the coming year.

January 1940

The Spring term started badly at Mortimer with outbreaks of 'flu', measles and food poisoning. This and the summer term progressed much as before with little evidence of hostilities, so that we lived in a fool's paradise and were completely unprepared, at least psychologically, for the horrendous events to reach us late in the year.

The new dental hospital opened in Lower Maudlin Street, opposite the old department at the Bristol Royal Infirmary (B.R.I.). Until then it had consisted of little more than a few rooms equipped with ancient dental chairs and few facilities, so that the new building was a revelation! There were something like thirty or more brand new modern dental chairs and units in the conservation room alone, together with well equipped laboratories, a lecture theatre, local and general anaesthetic rooms, prosthetic and orthodontic departments and a common room. To complete the picture was a basement kitchen for refreshments and a concrete air-raid shelter! (I think this became the inflammable store until 1980 when the danger of its proximity to canteen was realised- CDS)

The cricket season started in May at Coombe Dingle which was to become the venue for very many happy years, including my graduation from the second eleven to the 1st XI, my Secretaryship and Vice-Captain. All too good to be true until the "phoney war" came to an abrupt end on 10th May when Germany invaded Holland and Belgium. Neville Chamberlain resigned and our own Chancellor, Winston Churchill, replaced him as Prime Minister and War leader.

By the end of the Summer term these countries had surrendered and France had fallen with over 30 thousand British and colonial troops lost and 335 thousand successfully evacuated by an armada of little ships from Dunkirk back to these shores. We were issued with extensions to our gas masks and obliged to leave Mortimer House to make way for further "evacuees". These turned out to be King's College London women students - the final humiliation! The only consolation was that I managed to scrape through my 1st B.D.S. exam, but it was far from certain that there would be a University to return to by the end of the Summer vacation. A few weeks later I returned from holiday to register as a clinical student with the General Medical Council and started working at practical dental mechanics in the new hospital laboratory in July.

My quest for "digs" was soon fulfilled by joining several other dental students at a residence in Woodland Road, conveniently opposite the main University buildings and just up the road from the Princes Theatre. Several visits were made to the latter to see touring London shows, but unfortunately this was doomed to an early demise as a result of incendiary bombs, which completely gutted the place a few months later.[70]

A period of relative tranquility was soon to be shattered by air-raids from the German Luftwaffe over the City and especially targeting Filton Aeroplane Company, which was then one of the largest aeroplane manufacturing works in the world.

On one occasion whilst "fire-watching" on the roof of the new dental hospital at night, I witnessed the amazing sight of several barrage balloons going up in a blaze of fire, having been struck not by enemy action, but by lightning during a thunderstorm. During August and September, massive air-raids continued with high-explosive and incendiary bombs destroying the Rodney works at Filton. Casualties were heavy, as I witnessed first hand, since in addition to my A.R.P. (air-raid precaution) duties, I was now enrolled as a part-time stretcher-bearer at the B.R.I. This macabre atmosphere was heightened by my entry as an Anatomy student into the dissecting room where we had to share a cadaver in groups of four! Thankfully dental students limited their dissection to the head and neck!

The head of the department was Professor Whitnal and the dental tutor an elderly general practitioner by the name of Dr Stock, who seemed to suffer from perennial allergic rhinitis.

Physiology lectures were provided by the Dean of the Faculty of Medicine, Professor Brocklehurst, who always closed the theatre doors at 9.00 a.m. sharp to prevent the entry of late-comers. Histology practicals by Dr Thornton and experimental physiology (frogology!) and biochemistry by Dr Molly Wiltshire completed the picture, the latter's affliction seemed to be permanent indigestion! Having much later in life become an orthodontic lecturer myself, I can now more readily appreciate the effects that some students have on one's little idiosyncrasies!

November 1940

This particular month saw the first really serious interruption of our academic life with the start of the main blitz on the city itself from enemy aircraft.[71] On the Sunday evening of the 24th, all hell was let loose during a raid lasting from about 6.30 p.m. until 11.30 p.m. To quote from my diary:-"Bombs falling continuously. The worst hours I have ever experienced. Whistling bombs, parachute flares, incendiaries falling everywhere. Slight lull at 11.00 p.m. when I dashed down from my digs, where a large chunk of masonry had crashed through the sitting room window on to the table under which we were sheltering. I went to the B.R.I, where I was stretcher-bearing almost non-stop until nearly 7.00 a.m. the next morning. I saw several nasty operations in the theatre where surgeons Willway and Fitzgibbon were fully occupied, including several amputations. To quote the latter to us students - "This is not surgery, it's butchery!" Whilst lifting one elderly woman from the stretcher to the operating table her leg came away in my hands! The Anatomy department at the University is completely wrecked and the Great Hall has only its bare walls left standing. The tower is intact with a time-bomb (unexploded) alongside it. There is a terrible shortage of water owing to the pipe-lines being damaged and no gas.[72]

Tuesday 26th - woke up after a nap wondering if I had been dreaming. Fires are still burning, but Brocky (Professor Brocklehurst) still gave his lectures at 10.00 a.m. and 12.00 noon! There is a large bomb-crater between the old and new buildings.

A few days later we attended the Central Health Clinic for inoculation against typhoid fever and the same evening went to a lecture by Professor Rogers on "Trephining the Skull"! During the evening of 2nd December the next heavy air-raid started on the city lasting four hours, with stretcher bearing by candle-light, since the B.R.I, electricity

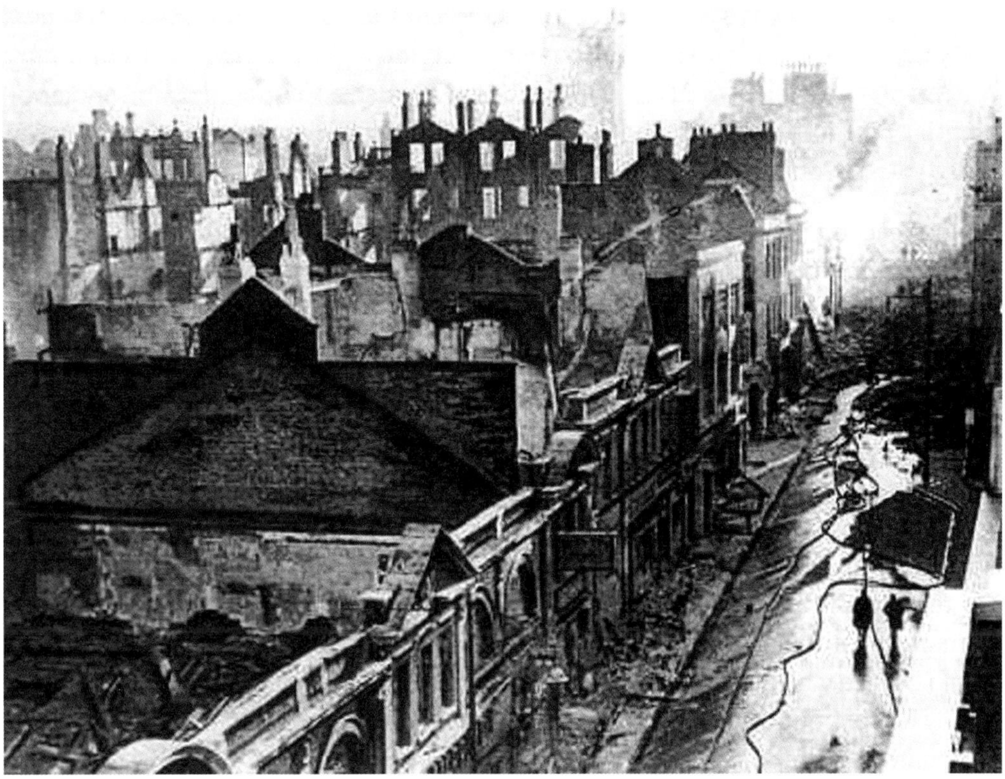

Figure 41. Union Street as it would have appeared to Hugh Leech on the morning of November 26th 1941 By kind permission of the Bristol Evening Post The whole area has now been replaced by the Broadmead shopping centre. The tower of St Peters church which remains as a memorial on Castle Park can just be seen through the smoke.

supply had failed.[73] This meant man-handling the stretchers to the operating theatres and wards around the defunct lift-shafts. The new library at the University was gutted and C Ward of the B.R.I. hit, with fortunately few casualties: likewise the Children's Hospital. Although our stretcher-bearing finished at 2.00 a.m., we still had to attend Prof's lecture at 9.00 a.m. with a film of William Harvey's description of the circulation of blood "De Motu Cordis"!

It was with a great sense of relief therefore that this momentous autumn term ended and I went down to the relative peace and quiet for a pleasant Christmas vacation.

January 1941

The air-raids continued throughout the first few months of the New Year, but dropped off gradually and life returned to the more normal. (*The raid of 7/8th May 1941 destroyed the roof of the nurse quarters of the Eye Hospital and also the mortuary of the BRI across the road so the Dental Hospital had two near misses- CDS*[74]).

The B.B.C. Symphony Orchestra, recently evacuated from London with its conductor

On the lighter side, the entertainment branch of their servicemen, the equivalent of our ENSA, put on a marvellous production of "This is the Army" at the Victoria Rooms stage with the renowned composer Irving Berlin writing, producing and acting in the show. The University "Revunions Society" was similarly active, but in not quite such a professional capacity and the more serious productions of the Dramatic Society were whole-heartedly supported, so that these activities were very good for the general morale during these trying times.

"Union Week" in June was an equally successful occasion starting with a "Biergarten" (beer being just about the only alcohol in sufficient quantity) and followed by garden parties at the halls of residence, the Senior Training Corps dance and several sports events. Having won our cricket match against King's College we later formed a combined XI to defeat the Welsh Universities handsomely. Our own dental team also beat the medicals, but again our combined efforts won the match against Thornbury on what was formerly the famous W. G. Grace's ground at Alveston, the opposing captain being none other than Dr. Grace, a more recent relative of the old man. One extraordinary event occurred as a result of this match being reported on the back sports page of our local newspaper, the Bristol Evening World. My brother, a signals officer attached to a regiment of the Somerset Yeomanry on active service in the Middle East, attended the field ablutions where the only hygienic essentials were provided by sheets of the flimsy overseas edition of this newspaper. Imagine his surprise when, prior to its use, he noticed his brother's name amongst the opening batsmen for the "Varsity". As usual the year closed with end-of-term exams, which in my case meant passing 1st Part Final B.D.S. Only one more to go.

1944

This final year started sadly with the death of Mr. Willway, who never suffered fools gladly, but whose teaching was universally admired, as was evident from the overflow of the congregation at his funeral in the B.R. I. chapel.

6th June was momentous for two reasons, one international and one personal. To quote from my diary

"Second Front opened at 6.00 a.m. Started my final exams! Paratroop, airborne and beach landings on the coast of Normandy between Le Havre and Cherbourg".

Soon afterwards final year medical students were commandeered to help with the returning casualties at Swindon and other hospitals. In September the "black-out" and fire-watching duties were abolished much to the tremendous universal relief. Sadly for us this meant the end of our accommodation at the B.R.I, as this was urgently required for the re-commissioning of new hospital wards.

Five of us were soon to be compensated by moving into a relatively palatial first floor flat (complete with grand piano, which I put to good use) and situated conveniently almost adjacent to Clifton Hill House Womens Hall of Residence! A very agreeable liaison with some of their residents resulted in our inviting them to an occasional Sunday lunch with an amicable arrangement - we provided the materials out of our food rations whilst they did the cooking. Washing-up was a mutual affair.

In December I mercifully completed my undergraduate training by passing my final B.D.S. exam and secured the post of acting unpaid junior house-surgeon at the dental hospital. Life was beginning to look very rosy, except that soon I would be eligible for call-up into His Majesty's services which filled me with no small amount of apprehension and excitement.

During the year several student weddings had taken place including that of a final year lady medical student to an American officer. Most of the reception was provided by the U.S. Forces, which was a revelation to guests who had long suffered the deprivation of war-time austerity. I have a vague recollection of new dustbins filled with ice and bottles of rum and coco-cola!

The December Dental Students Dance at the Victoria Rooms was a great success with our special guests in attendance - "Percy" Stoy (Dean), Georgie Fawn (Dental Surgery), Trevor Johnson (Orthodontics), Claremont (Periodontology) and Pickles (Prosthetics). These were the teachers who had tolerated us for so long and coerced us through our exams.

1945

My final few months at the start of this new year continued to be full of interest, not least of which was the visit of our Chancellor himself, Winston Churchill, who conferred honorary degrees in the University Great Hall on Ernest Bevin (Minister of Labour) and A. V. Alexander (Defence Minister). "Winnie" as he was affectionately known looked very tired to those of us acting as ushers, which was not surprising considering his strenuous war years as War Leader and Prime Minister. This appearance, however, disguised his real mental state which was as active as ever, judging by the delivery of his usual masterly speech.

Victory in Europe

V. E. Day, was announced by him in May and at the end of the Spring term I very sadly went down from this wonderful university for good. Within a month I had been called up into the Army Dental Corps as a 2nd Lieutenant for preliminary training at York barracks, and then Aldershot. This seemed to me a little pointless now that the war in Europe was finally over. However, there was still the war to be waged against Japan which looked as if it would continue for some considerable time with many more casualties. Mercifully this was brought to a rapid conclusion following the dropping of atomic bombs on Hiroshima and Nagasaki. My anticipated involvement in the "real war" was therefore never to materialise.

After the preliminary few months army training I was posted as a dental officer to the Parachute Training Depot at Hardwick Hall in Derbyshire. Having been foolhardy enough to volunteer to do my jumps, I was thankfully turned down on medical reasons, purely because I wore spectacles! Previously recruits were rejected if they wore full dentures, even though they were otherwise 100 fit. This was because of the risk of swallowing them or choking during the impact of landing! A simple solution was found by my dental predecessors who designed metal denture containers into which the teeth were to be placed just prior to leaving the aircraft. Needless to say, many airmen used them as tobacco pouches instead!

Many of those I met and treated were wonderful battle-hardened men, but even so there were one or two who said they would rather be back at Arnhem than visit my surgery! A memorable sight each morning was the batman polishing the artificial leg of the officer in the billet next to mine - the human original having been blown off previously in action. It was with an element of regret and eager anticipation that I left this unit after a year and was posted to the canal zone in Egypt. The following two years were also full of adventure and fulfilment prior to my eventual "demob" in 1948, but that is another story.

Afterthoughts

Except during the periods of direct enemy action, most students, like their other young contemporaries, enjoyed themselves to the full. "Eat, drink and be merry, for tomorrow... etc".

Food was sufficient and even the powdered egg and milk and ubiquitous "spam" (tinned ham) were tolerated after a while. Fresh food was limited and fresh fruit only available during the normal British season, since imports from abroad were severely restricted. I remember the look of incredulity on the face of a small patient at the B.R.I, children's ward who was completely nonplussed by the nature and purpose of the present given to him by an American G.I. serviceman. It was a banana. He had never seen one before!

Special functions such as weddings and birthday parties required some ingenuity, the "banquet" often consisting of vegetable soup, fresh chicken (no home freezers then) and tinned fruit pudding, for which ration coupons had to be sacrificed. Ice cream was often unobtainable and I remember some American servicemen friends motoring by jeep all the way to Blackpool especially to find some, after seeing holiday makers there enjoying it, as shown on the Pathe cinema news. Practically the only celebratory alcohol consisted of sherry, Algerian wine and beer. Whisky, gin and other spirits were in extremely short supply and usually only obtainable "under the counter".

There were no bars at the Coombe Dingle Sports ground, so that celebratory drinking or otherwise took place at the Victoria Rooms where the visiting teams were entertained.

Fairly weak Georges Bristol Bitter Beer was the only drink available. Mixed company usually retired to "Aunties", the nearest local pub run by two elderly ladies and very popular with both students and Americans. For non-alcoholic beverages, Fortes Ice-Cream Parlour and the Berkeley Cafe opposite the university were popular, as was the Blackboy cafe near the Clifton Downs.

Horts and The Grand Hotel were reserved for special occasions for those of us who could afford them. This usually meant supplementing our meagre parental allowances (few University grants then) by paid fire-watching on the roofs of such places as Harvey's Wine cellars at 10 shillings per night. The greater attraction of earning £5 per night on the fuel dumps at Avonmouth docks was left to the more patriotic and foolhardy!

For more up-market entertainment, Bristol was very fortunate in that the tragic destruction of the city from air-raids did not affect such places as the Colston Hall, the Theatre Royal and the Hippodrome, where symphony concerts, classical plays and the performances of visiting Opera companies took place.

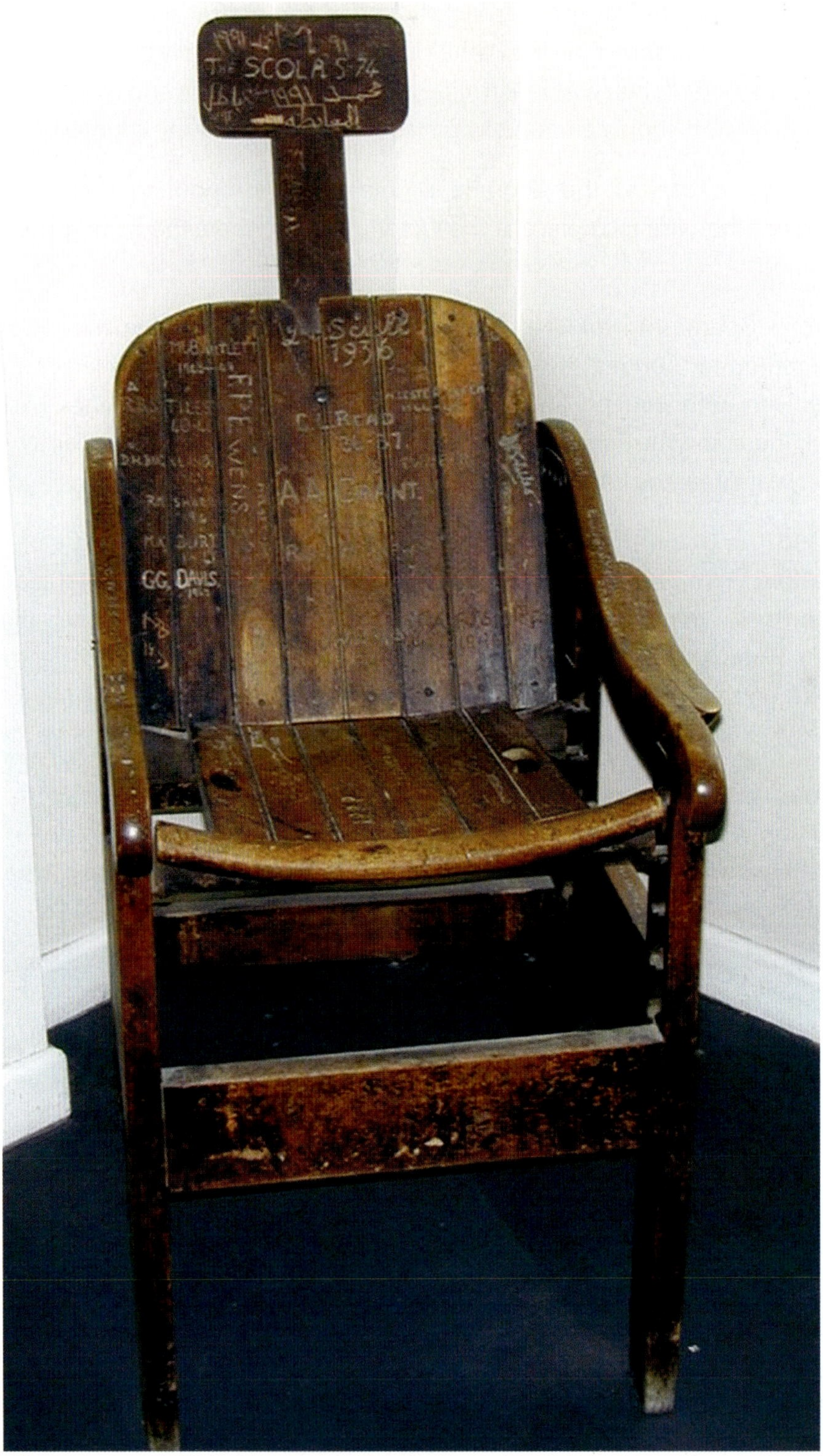

Figure 43. The Bristol dental chair.

CHAPTER 6

THE BRISTOL DENTAL CHAIR

The only artefact of any historic significance held in the Bristol Dental School is a dental chair. It is of entirely wooden construction in which the height of the seat and headrest can be adjusted.

Quite when the chair was acquired and who bought it has been a matter for conjecture for some time as there is no record of its origin.

The Bristol General Hospital was the first to establish a post specific to dentistry when in 1874 the position of Surgeon Dentist was created and Thomas Cooke Parsons elected to it. Six years later the General Hospital was also the first to establish a "Special Department of Dental Surgery".

The Bristol Infirmary (later the Bristol Royal Infirmary) continued to expect dental procedures to be part of the duties of the general surgeon until 1888 when it opened its Dental Department and appointed William Robert Ackland as their Dental Surgeon. Before he came to Bristol, at the age of 25, Ackland had been Demonstrator of Practical Dental Surgery at the Dental Hospital of London which by this time had moved to Leicester Square. One of his colleagues there was the 42 year old Charles Sissmore Tomes FRS, son of Sir John Tomes, who was already an examiner for the LDSRCS Eng. It is interesting to note that in the year Ackland was appointed in Bristol Claudius Ash and Sons donated £500 towards the extension of the Dental Hospital of London.[75] Clearly the company had seen the commercial wisdom of supporting charitable institutions dedicated to dental education and it is just possible that they may have sponsored the Bristol dental chair.

The BDA have a very similar chair in the museum collection dating from about 1860. The Bristol model does not appear in a 1860s catalogue but does in the 1886 Ash catalogue (*page 80*) which was made primarily for charitable institutions. The only difference is the more rudimentary head rest of the Bristol model which may well be a replacement. The improved chair mentioned in the advertisement above was probably the considerably more sophisticated model which had been exhibited by George Owen LDSRCS Eng of the North London Dental Dispensary at the meeting of the Odontological Society in December 1858.[76]

being appointed two years later as a dental mechanic at a salary of £325 p.a. In due course he was to become Chief Technician and Dental Instructor, a post he served with great distinction for many years until his retirement in 1982. He will be remembered by generations of students for his lilting Welsh voice coming through the public address system in the prosthetics laboratory. The familiar "Can I have your attention please?" was always preceded by two puffs into the microphone.

A further significant development in 1947 was the agreement with the BRI surgeons that there could now be one male and one female bed in the Infirmary given over to dental in-patients. There would also be a Resident Dental House Officer seconded to the BRI from one of the Dental Hospital posts.[86]

The Schools Dental Service had started as a privately funded venture in Cambridgeshire in 1907. The Bristol Central Health Clinic, which was to be the centre of operations for the city's School Dental Service, opened in 1937. The service remained under local authority control after the NHS Act of 1948 but agreement had already been reached by this time for the Dental Hospital to be responsible for the dental care of two Bristol schools in order to provide suitable teaching experience for students.[87] Before long, school children started coming to the Dental Hospital in large numbers and four cubicles were provided for them in the Conservation Room.

In most universities the academic head of a dental school is called "Dental Dean" or "Dean of Dental Studies". However the Bristol Dental School had been established at a time when dentistry was run by a Dental Board of the General Medical Council on which sat a medically qualified dental representative, it was therefore logical for the head of the school in Bristol to be seen as an assistant dean to the Dean of the Medical Faculty. Mr PJ Stoy, who had been appointed in 1934 as the first full-time dental lecturer in dental mechanics, was made Dental Assistant Dean to the Dean of the Faculty of Medicine in 1940, that is to say a Dean of Dental Studies in all but name. When the School of Veterinary Science opened in 1948 Bristol became the only university with three integrated clinical schools and it seemed logical for the same arrangement to operate in what became known as the "Bristol System" where the day to day running of each school was organised by an assistant dean. Eventually there were to be six such deans with the addition of a preclinical dean in each school.

When in 1947, Arthur I Darling was brought to the University by the then Vice-Chancellor, Sir Philip Morris it was logical that he should be in charge of teaching and so was appointed as "Director of Dental Studies". This required no change in the running of the Medical Faculty and Stoy, who had done so much to set up the new school remained, as Dental Assistant Dean and was responsible for its the day to day running. This was an advantage for Professor Darling who could get now get on with developing research in the school. Almost immediately though the popular Philip Stoy left to become Professor of Dental Surgery and later Dean of the Belfast Dental School [88] much to the dismay of the students[89] for Percy as he was known was much loved and excellent teacher.

According to Professor DC Berry when first appointed Arthur Darling's blunt North-country approach did not go down at all well. "He sang Geordie' songs at Dental School concerts and, anyway, he was far too young to be a Professor."[90] There was opposition too from some of the part-time honorary dental surgeons and senior members of the Medical Faculty who looked on him as a young upstart.

The then dental students, many of them ex–servicemen, were not amused to find on entering their clinical studies "down the road" that gowns now had still to be worn in lectures (Arthur Darling insisted on this until the early 1970s) and that beards were to be removed. A further change was that no student was permitted to take the LDSRCS examination of a Royal College unless they had sat the BDS Bristol at least once.

George Fawn, who had done much to bring about the establishment of the School also retired in 1947. To quote Professor Darling himself

> *... there can be little doubt that with the resignation of Mr George Fawn in 1947 an era at the Dental Hospital ended. He epitomised the "visiting honorary". Full of the wisdom of long practice, with an unending flow of stories of earlier days, he was loved and respected by every student as well as by his colleagues. On his retirement, the staff and students of the Dental Hospital contributed £100 (then half the cost of a small family saloon car- CDS) to commemorate his long and valuable service and the George Fawn Prize was instituted. "*[91]

He continued to practice at 6 Oakfield Road, Bristol at least until 1954 and lived there until his death in the early 1970s at the age of 83 years.

The coming of the National Health Service

During the discussions and negotiations with the Ministry of Health on the new National Health Service Act, it was important to have a body that could speak for the entire profession. At this time under the Articles of the BDA dental practitioners registered under Dentists Act of 1921 with no registrable qualification were excluded from membership. This long-standing difficulty was resolved when, in January 1947, members attending an Extraordinary General Meeting of the Association voted to cancel this Article thus paving the way, in December 1949, for the amalgamation of the Incorporated Dental Society and the Public Dental Service Association with the BDA. In his book "The Western Counties Branch of the British Dental Association"

Alexander Woods wrote:

> *'Beyond doubt it was in the minds of many that complete amalgamation could not be effected by the simple process of passing a resolution in London. It was to be at branch and section levels that professional esprit de corps would be developed and focussed. During this epoch making period the branch was again fortunate in its Honorary Secretary, Robert Hunt. His agreeable personality, tact, and energy were at their best in the negotiations and arrangements that culminated in amalgamation.'*[92]

Hunt subsequently became President of the Western Counties Branch in 1959 and served as a member and as chairman of a number of BDA committees and in 1967 was elected Chairman of the Representative Board.

A start was made in 1948 in providing consultant services in those areas of the country where they were deficient. Paying consultants the same throughout the country whatever their speciality helped in this process. The concept of a District Hospital (a local hospital serving a natural geographic area) was adopted by the NHS. This decision went back many years to the Dawson Report (1920). Such hospitals were coupled with university hospitals where more complex facilities were available.

Proposals were drafted the following year for the DentalHospital to provide orthodontic services for all Bristol children and a full-time orthodontist became necessary. This was to be Bill Nicol who on demobilisation from the Army Dental Corps in 1945 had undertaken his orthodontic training at the Royal Dental Hospital. He came to Bristol in 1948 and initially worked under the honorary Trevor Johnson before becoming a full time NHS consultant in 1957. From then until 1966 he carried the full load of orthodontic teaching and at the same time was responsible for treatment of patients referred by the Schools Dental Service.

Among the many bodies set up by the government in 1943 in anticipation of the NHS was the Teviot committee. Its interim report of 1944 had recommended that any National Health Service should include a comprehensive dental service and its final report of 1945 warned that the UK needed many more dentists than could possibly be trained with the available facilities. The end of the War in 1945 and the return of the ex-servicemen saw the dental schools filled as never before but by 1950 the ex-servicemen were fewer and more candidates for dental education were needed.

With the arrival of the NHS the Dental Management Committee now became the Joint Management Committee of the Dental Hospital which embraced Hospital and University inputs. It first met on 4th November 1948 and from then on was invariably chaired by the Vice Chancellor Sir Philip Morris. It reported to the Dental Sub Committee of the Medical Board of the University.

Teaching staff at this time were:

a) Dental Surgery

Professor A. I. Darling (Head)
L. E. Claremont (Dental Materia Medica)
D.C.Connor
R.J.Fowler
D. Gibson Davies
P.M.Nicholas
S.K.Rigg
R.S.Saxton
NH Simmonds (Dental Radiology)
J.W.E. Snawdon

b) Dental Prosthetics

A.O.Chick
F.R.Hogbin
J.Wells

c) Childrens Dentistry

W.T.Johnson (Orthodontics, and Head)
L.E.Claremont
W.A.Nicol

It is interesting to see that children's dentistry was a separate department at this time, probably because its contractual commitment to provide treatment for school children. It was noted that in that year 1900 children had been registered, 500 orthodontic plates fitted and 1300 gas cases seen. Dental Surgery was much larger than the other two departments because it included dental medicine and oral surgery and therefore did the bulk of the teaching.

Changes now came thick and fast. Immediately it was decided to abolish the fees for the student dental attendants (later known as dental surgery assistants or dental nurses).This was because it had proved impossible to collect them! This was hardly surprising since at 20 guineas their fees were almost a quarter of their annual pay of £83-8s 4d![93] The same meeting agreed that the Dental Hospital could be used for evening classes in dental mechanics (dental technology) to be given by the Merchant Venturers Technical College which was still in existence at this time. A few months later it was decided that the University would pay for the Dental Hospital's own technicians to attend this College's City and Guilds course.

Serious efforts had been made to popularise dentistry as a career, as a result, by 1955 or thereabouts, there was a steadily increasing demand for entry into the dental schools. Many factors were instrumental in effecting this change, of which the Willink Report on Medicine (1957) and the McNair Report on Dentistry (1956) were undoubtedly important. Perhaps more important still was the tremendous increase in the demand for higher education. By 1950, as services expanded in the Dental Hospital space was becoming a problem, but the first real discussion of an extension to the Dental Hospital was raised following a request from the UGC in 1950 to increase the dental intake by 50%[94]. At the same meeting in October of that year the decision was taken to appoint the Hospital's first dental hygienist but there was some delay in making an appointment. Miss K.M.E Griffiths finally took this up on 1st April 1951.

Following detailed discussions with the Governors of the United Bristol Hospitals agreement was reached for establishing a 2 year training programme for dental attendants which would be funded by the United Bristol Hospitals, and 7 students started the course in 1951. Sister Dawes resigned in 1952 and for the next 23 years Sister Davidson (Sybil Moores) was in charge of dental nursing. At the time of writing she still maintains her interest in the School at the age of 99 years. The course soon proved very popular and gave the Hospital the opportunity of filling any vacancy with the best of those who qualified each year who were then paid £4-0-0 per week!.

There was now a national need for more suitably trained dental teaching staff. This was not surprising in a profession expanding at such a rate. Staff were difficult to find for they were drawn from the much smaller student output of the recent past. There was also often a shortage of funds. It should be remembered that the country was dealing with the economic consequences of the war. Many resources were scarce and rationing did not finally end until 1953. Finally there were the financial attractions of general dental practice in the early days of the NHS. In spite of these difficulties the number of staff slowly increased.

Up to this time the hospital and school produced most of their own junior staff from among their graduates and, in spite of a healthy exchange of staff at higher levels, approximately half of the staff were "Bristol trained". Jim Fletcher (BDS U Brist, 1951) became a lecturer in 1959. A second chair was created that year (5 years after it had first been discussed) and filled by Eric Bradford who became Professor of Dental Surgery and now took over the running of dental conservation. Arthur Darling's title was changed to that of Professor of Oral Medicine. David Berry who finished his national service with the RAF and qualified from Bristol in 1949 was appointed as a lecturer soon afterwards but resigned in July 1953.[95] He would be reappointed in 1960 and soon became responsible for dental prosthetics although he did not receive his chair in dental prosthetics until much later.

Mr. J W Ross, was appointed in November 1963 to replace Mr. Snawdon in Oral Surgery Earlier the same year Mr. JC (Chris) Stephenson became the first NHS consultant to hold a linked hospital appointment with 2 days at Bath and the remainder at the Dental Hospital. This orthodontic post and a series of later hospital appointments linked the School to local regional dental units with considerable mutual benefit.

By 1962 the total number of dental students in the school was 138 and the staff numbered approximately 20 full-time and 9 part-time. During the period 1949-1962 the annual out-patient attendances at the Hospital increased from 31,755 to 65,317.

The undergraduate course

In the late 1940s students still undertook their 2nd BDS anatomy and physiology studies with the medical students in the old anatomy department in University Road. Human dissection was an important component for all clinical students. The Professor of Physiology endeared himself to the students by arriving on the dot and then locking the door so no late comers could enter the lecture. Dental anatomy lectures were given in the dental school on Saturday mornings.

Having passed 2nd BDS there was then a year of dental mechanics. Prosthetic technique teaching was under the charge of Sidney Mattock although Ivor Robinson and Dobbie Dobson were now also on the scene, (Dobbie arrived in 1949 and would remain there until his retirement as Chief Instructor in January 1988). All the craft elements (lots of

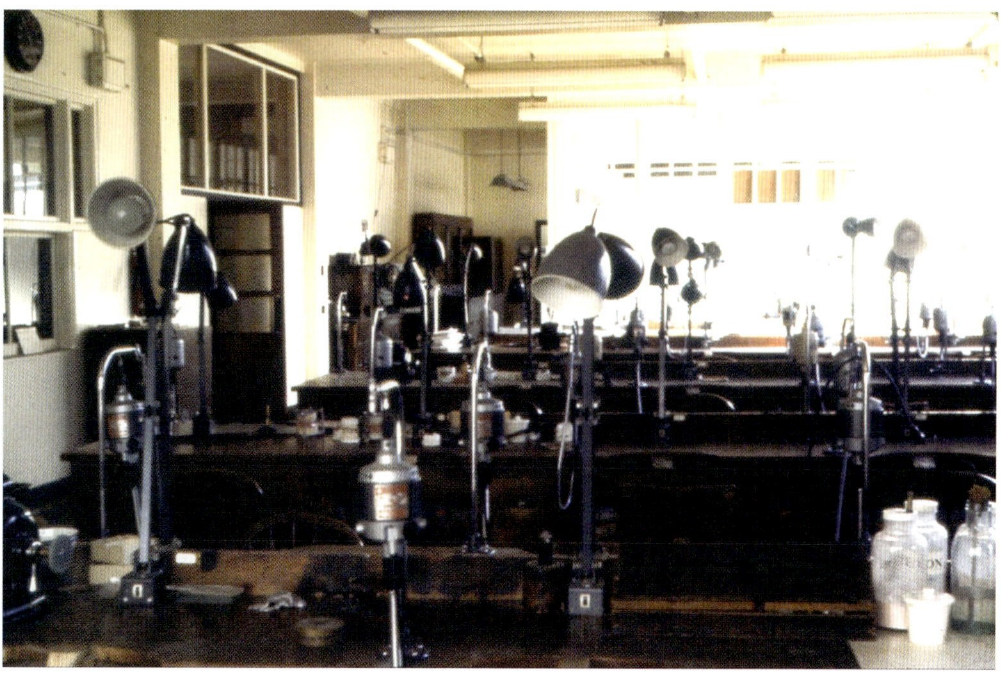

Figure 49. The 1940 Dental Mechanics Laboratory, later known as the Prosthetics teaching lab.

soldering, casting, swaging and trial set ups) which dental schools later abandoned were still taught on the technique course and students would then undertake all their own technical work for patients. Vulcanite was on the way out but plaster impressions were still used for full dentures with alginate reserved for partial dentures.

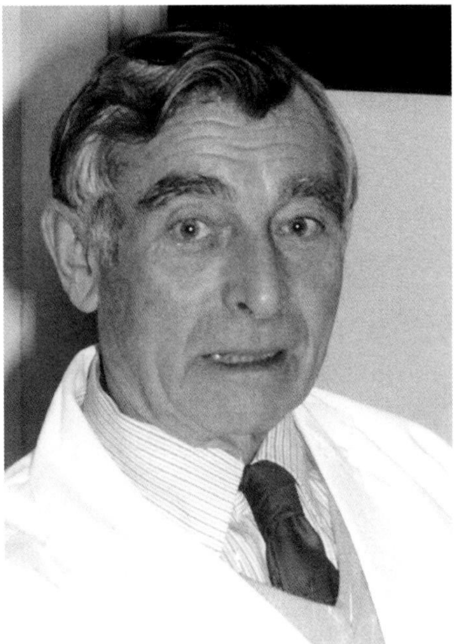

Figure 50. Dobbie Dobson, Chief Dental Instructor on his retirement in 1988.

The operative technique course in conservative dentistry then followed with cohesive gold still being used. In oral surgery students administered their own general anaesthesics under the watchful eye of the remarkable Professor Tratman who had by now returned from the Singapore Dental School. It was said of Trat that dentistry was his profession but spelaeology was his life.[96] The story is told that when Singapore was about to be overrun by the Japanese he hid the dental gold in the schools' water tanks and was able to retrieve this when he returned there after the war.

A visit by members of the University Grants Committee in February 1947 was unanimous in its view that the school was well equipped and could accommodate more students.[97] The dental intake thereafter gradually increased from 18 to 25 By 1957 there was again pressure, this time from the Medical Faculty Board, for a further increase to 35 students. It was realised that before this could happen additional clinical space would be required and planning for what would become the 1964 extension began. The undergraduate course was changing to make room for including the scientific basis of dentistry. There was more time allocated for private study and lectures became optional rather than obligatory in many subjects. There was the beginning of what later became known as " whole patient care" where students carried out work according to the patients needs rather than complete quotas of clinical work in each department. Presentation of a selection of these cases , which became known as "Final fives" was a crucial part of the final examination.

A cause of great distress during this period was the untimely death in 1961 of John Snawdon, who was the youngest of the "honoraries" and a most gifted member of the staff. He took a close interest in the hospital and its students and served as Dental Assistant Dean. But apart from his clinical skills he is remembered by those who were students at this time for his tremendous work in beginning and running the students' annual reunion. After his departure it gradually declined until abandoned in the mid 1970s.

The 1964 Extension

In 1957 the new Dentists Act had given autonomy to the dental profession which was no longer merely a dental board of the General Medical Council. As a result, dentistry became responsible for its own standards of education although doctors still retained the right to practise dentistry without any additional training! The enthusiasm of the new General Dental Council, together with the report of the McNair Committee, eventually convinced government that more places were needed in dental schools and the process of expansion was begun.

The enlargement of the Bristol Dental Hospital and School, so long awaited was begun in August 1961. The planning sub committee for this had in fact been set up in October 1950. Then it consisted of Arthur Darling, Trevor Johnson, John Snawdon and Professor Bruce Perry with the University Secretary Evan Wright in attendance. At first the possibility of using two adjacent shops or building over the car park at the rear were considered, but it was soon realised that a much larger site would be needed. This was achieved by extending up Lower Maudlin Street and around the corner into Upper Maudlin Street. It involved the loss of the Prince Alfred pub, greatly regretted by students and some staff.* The final building doubled the size of the School and provided for an increase in the annual intake of students from twenty-five a year to fifty a year.

The architects for the new building were Watkins, Orey and Partners and the first stage of the project, the building of the extension itself, was completed in June 1963. The second stage involved the modification of the "old building", and was completed in March 1964. The cost of the building was £350,000.[98] Furniture and equipment cost another £110,000 which was paid for by the Ministry of Health. The student intake was increased to 35 in October 1963 and then to 50 in October 1964, after the completion of the entire project.

It is interesting to read the notes of the planning meeting for the new building. As so much of the new building concerned the teaching of restorative dentistry it was logical that Professor Bradford would take the lead. This also explains why he would include his own small laboratory and private lavatory. The only exception to this general plan might appear to be the so called "Histopathogy Laboratory" which

---

* The suggestion that a certain member of staff was occasionally seen emerging from the pub at 9.00 a.m. to walk the short distance to the Dental School is hotly denied!

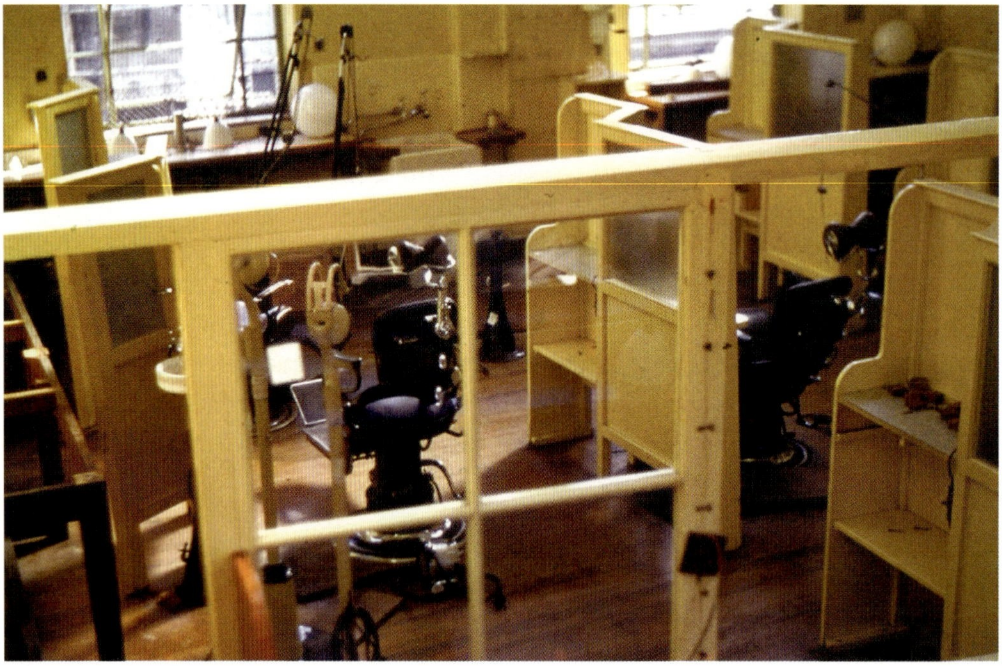

Figure 51. Equipment in the Prosthetics Department in 1959 showing the 1948 DMCo chairs.

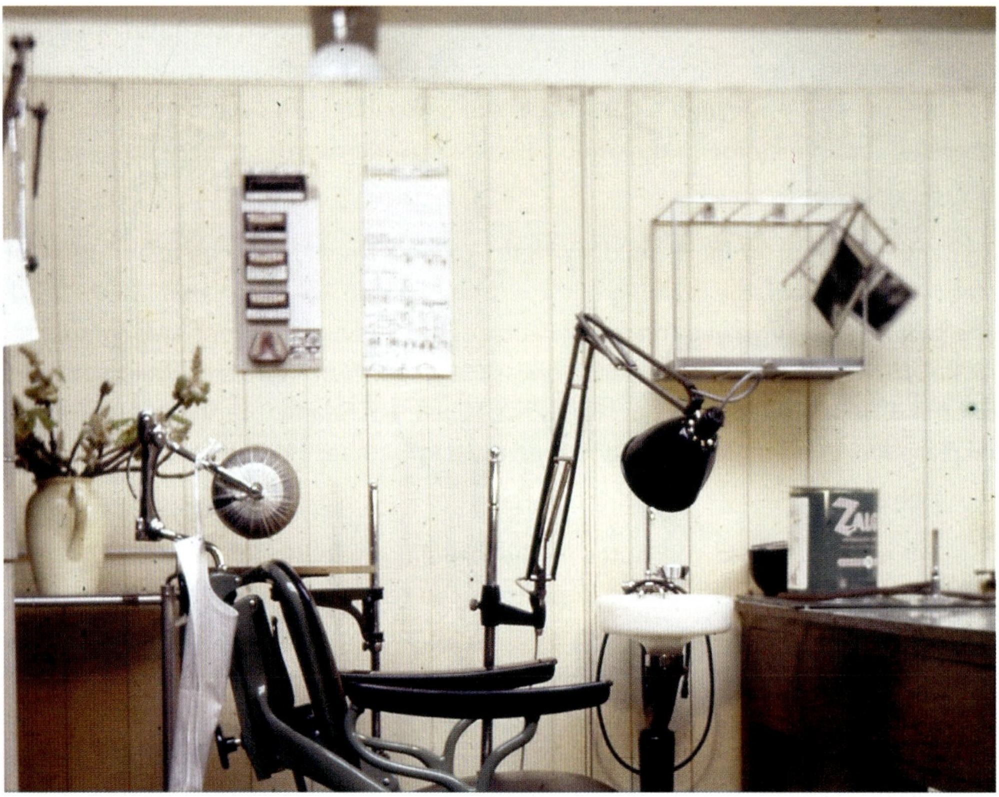

Figure 52. Similar equipment in the orthodontic department - note the large tin of Zelgan alginate!

occupied the greater part of one side of the building on the 1st floor. In fact this was planned as a phantom head room as Eric Bradford had always felt it was desirable to have this on the same floor and close to the conservation chairs. It was his hope that when technique courses were not running individual students could practice their conservation techniques; for example when a patient had cancelled an appointment at short notice. However a late inclusion in the planning committee minutes was the agreement to a proposal by Arthur Darling that when not in use for technique courses this large area might be used by other departments. By the 1970's the Oral Medicine Department was the main user of this large space and on Wednesday mornings 50 microscopes were duly set out. For the rest of the week the room was largely unused except to store students, conservation kits.

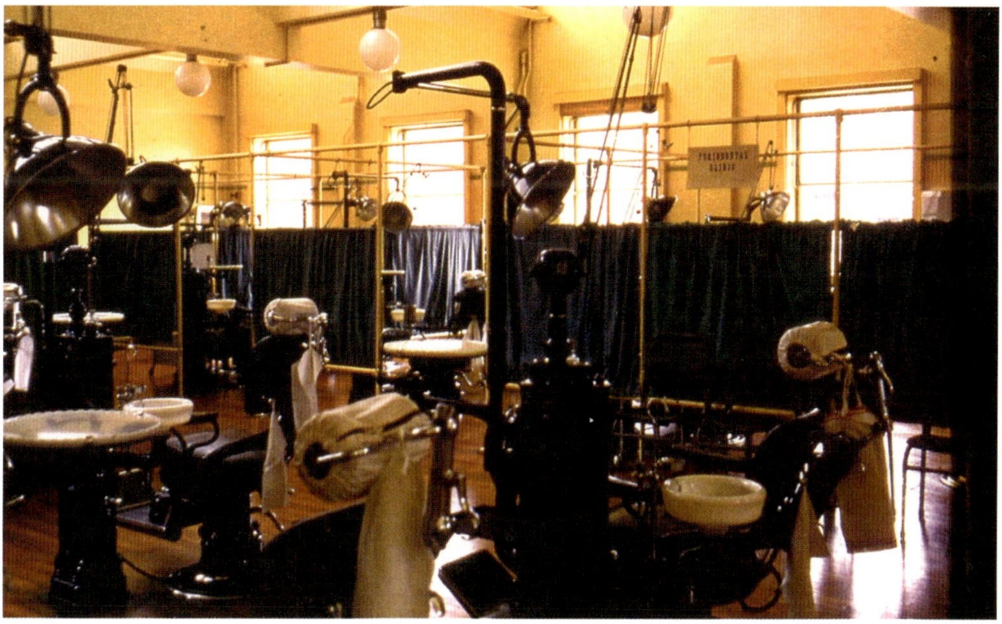

Figure 53. The old conservation department before the opening of the new extension.- no air-rotors!

Research

As Dr David Poole's obituary for Professor Darling says:

> *"Arthur Darling, however, was never happier than when he was involved in research. Almost as soon as he had arrived in Bristol, he had laid the foundations for developing a research element in the school. The perennial problem of shortage of funds led to his seeking of support from the Medical Research Council..."*

In fact one of his first actions after his appointment in 1948 was to get agreement from the Dental Committee for the conversion of the operating theatre in the Dental Hospital to a research laboratory. His first recruits to this were two young zoology graduates Mary Hay and Audrey Fisher who were engaged in the tissue culture of developing teeth. Later with the addition of David Poole and Maurice Stack the work expanded to include the study of the structure and chemistry of teeth . This small team was soon joined by two members of clinical staff, Stuart Crabb and David Lyon, for whom research became a passion. This expanding team was accommodated with difficulty in extremely cramped quarters on the first floor of the 1939 dental school building where currently the waiting room for the Department of Child Dental Health is sited.

In 1961 the group became the MRC Dental Research Unit, under the direction of Arthur Darling. It was only the second MRC Research Unit to be created and the only one in existence at that time (the first in London having been closed down). The remit of the unit was to attempt to solve the problem of dental caries, then seen as the major cause of dental disease, but it also afforded a valuable opportunity for future members of staff to get some experience of basic research and acted as an important stimulus to the staff and students of the hospital and school. Together with the work being carried on in Arthur's own department, the wider research interests of the school attracted an international reputation. This changing emphasis was reflected nationally. The British Division of the International Association for Dental Research was established in 1953 and held its inaugural meeting on 21st March that year at Guy's Hospital.

Although the expansion in student numbers in 1961-4 was reflected in increased numbers of staff in the hospital and its academic departments, it was observed and regretted by Professor Darling that relatively few of them saw much career advantage by spending time on research. This was not surprising. At the time clinical academic posts, unlike those of the university generally, were linked to NHS hospital training rather than to research output. There was no prospect of being advanced to consultant senior lecturer without fulfilling the Royal College's requirement for consultant status and so, for a young clinical academic, the completion of their specialist training was their first priority. Appointments committees for consultant senior lecturer posts always included a College representative and the first duty of the chairman of such a committee was to ask the representative formally if all the candidates about to be interviewed fulfilled the College's requirements. Those who did not could only be appointed on the lecturer scale and would have to accept a lower honorary NHS status and work under the supervision of a consultant. At this time it was only after having achieved consultant status that the academic turned his or her attention to gaining a higher degree by research. As specialist training become longer and College requirements more stringent this focus on research might be deferred until much later, perhaps in the trainees middle thirties. In due course this conflict was recognised and partially solved by centrally funded fixed term posts designed to enable the appointee to fulfil both a research doctorate and completion of specialist training during a period with very limited teaching duties.

In 1965 Professor Darling turned his attention to the basic sciences and acquired funding for a chair in oral biology with associated lectureships in anatomy physiology and biochemistry. It was expected that Dr David Poole, who had been working very productively in the MRC Dental Research Unit at Bristol, would be promoted but to everyone's surprise Dr Declan Anderson from Guys was appointed. The following is quoted from the latter's interview in 1992 with H Colin Davies published after Arthur's death.[99]

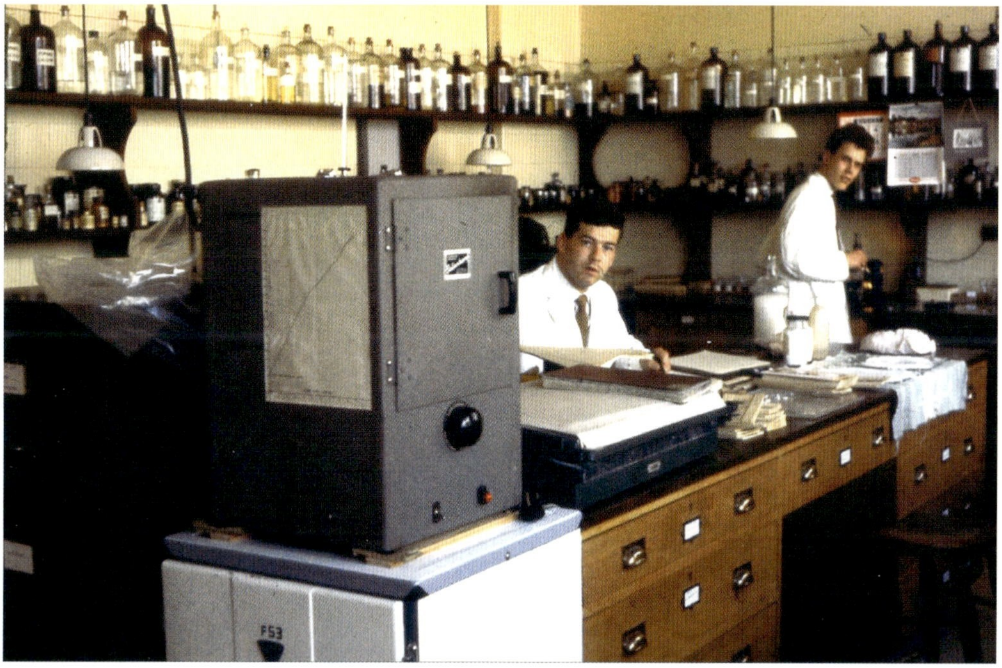

Figure 54. Equipment in the Prosthetics Department in 1959 showing the 1948 DMCo chairs.

DA... it looked as though it (his appointment to Bristol) might bridge the preclinical clinical divide. Also I was tired of commuting to London and I wanted to get away from academic strife.

HCD A pious hope surely. I suppose Darling was one of the last old style Deans, the equivalent of robber barons ***l'etat c'est moi*** and all that . Wasn't it said of him "he was sometimes wrong but never in doubt"?

DA We certainly had mammoth battles but never lost our respect for each other: We frequently broke off for lunch in the senior common room where we would arrive shouting at each other. I think our colleagues expected it of us and they were seldom disappointed.

CHAPTER 8

TIMES OF CHANGE AND UNCERTAINTY 1972-1989

The year of 1971, which saw Arthur Darling receiving the CBE in the New Year's Honours list, also saw the creation and filling of 2 new UGC funded lectureships in periodontology and orthodontics. This was to mark the end of earmarked UGC grants for dentistry and university expansion in general for many years. By this time so severe was the pressure for extra accommodation in the school that Professor Eric Bradford persuaded the University to rent 1500 sq ft of office space on the second floor of a commercially owned building. The space in Priory House (later Manulife House) in Marlborough Street, was used for laboratories and staff rooms.[100] This building was demolished in 2001 to make way for the University's Dorothy Hodgkin Research Building.

In the late 1960s the Wellcome Trust had been persuaded by Arthur Darling to fund the building of a research wing at a cost of £198,946. There was considerable delay while the City Archaeologist carried out detailed excavation of the site as described in

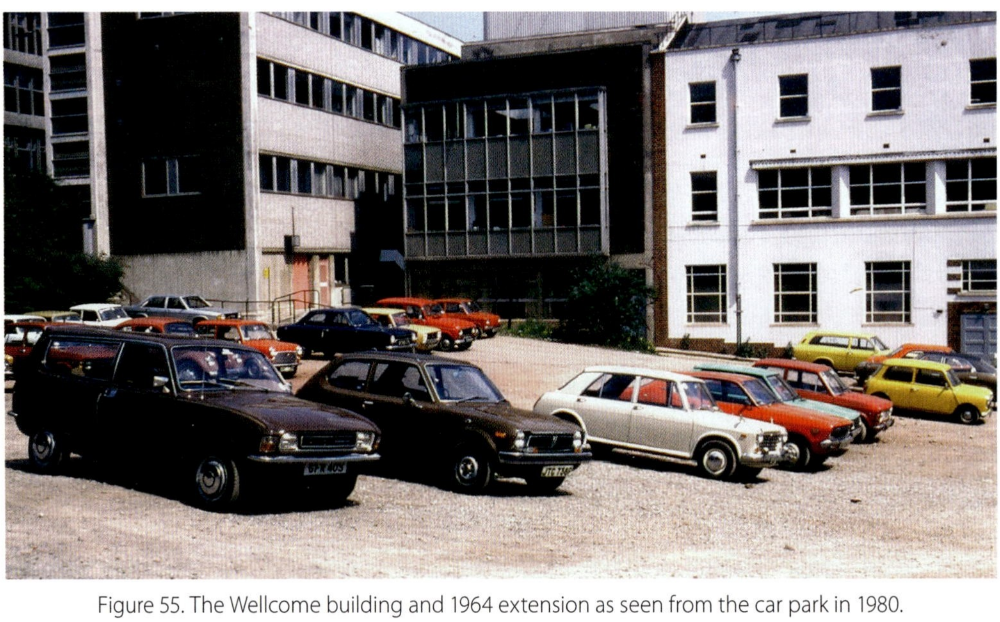

Figure 55. The Wellcome building and 1964 extension as seen from the car park in 1980.

Chapter 1. Building work finally started in March 1974 and was completed in June 1975. The architects were Eustace H Button and Partners who would go on to design further buildings for the School . The new wing was owned by the University but the majority of the space was rented by the MRC for its Dental Research Unit with approximately 350 square metres being reserved for the University. This allowed the Dental Research Unit to continue to grow until 25 staff were accommodated there. The Unit made a valuable contribution to the School not only in research but also in teaching of the biological sciences.

This increase in research and laboratory accommodation did little to relieve the growing need for further space in all clinical areas. Much of this was due to the need to comply with the new GDC directive: to teach low seated "4 handed" dentistry. This greatly increased the footprint of every dental chair and required adjacent cabinetry so that all materials and instruments were in reach of the student rather than obtained centrally. Further pressure came from the need to provide space for the new Dental Hygiene School which had opened with 6 trainees in 1972 under the Directorship of Marsh Midda who was also Consultant in Periodontology. A year after his appointment Marsh was being pressed by the Department of Health to double the Hygiene School intake.

Technician training was becoming formalised with a proper career structure and in conjunction with the Area Health Authority a Technical Training Course was set up to ensure a steady supply of qualified dental technicians. This solved the problem of filling technical vacancies with appropriately trained staff. Finally there was the wish to introduce a fully integrated longitudinal course in restorative skills. This was impossible because the school was unique in the UK in having only one technique laboratory which had to be adapted three times a year to run either prosthetic or on one of the two conservation technique courses. Thus the School was wedded to block teaching in these two subjects.

The Conservatives had swept to power in 1970 and Sir Keith Joseph, who was appointed Secretary of State for Social Services with a particular responsibility for the National Health Service, believed that the growing problem of the NHS could be resolved solely by reforming its management structure. He was not the first nor the last to hold such views and quite failed to appreciate that it would merely increase expenditure on bureaucracy without the corresponding improvement in quality of service. (Joseph was later said to be appalled by the monster he had created and came to the conclusion that he had concentrated too much on management and too little on philosophy.)

The White Paper outlining the Government's proposals was published in August 1972 and these came into effect in 1973. The result of the White Paper was the abolition of the old Board of Governors of the United Bristol Hospitals and their incorporation into a three layered administration. The local hospitals became part of the Bristol Health District (Teaching) which had its headquarters in Manulife House, in Marlborough Street. This reported to the Avon Area Authority which had theirs in the newly built Whitefriars building Lewin's Mead and above was the SW Regional Health Authority which was based in King Square. The one good thing for Bristol dentistry in this complex hierarchy was that the able and charismatic Tom Dowell became the Area Dental Officer "with Regional responsibilities" . Later he would be formally appointed as the Regional Dental Officer. With the support of Gordon Tucker as his District Dental Officer Tom set about integrating Hospital and Community Dental Services to the great benefit of the Dental Hospital and School. He and his colleagues organised and ran a new Dental Public Health course for undergraduates which opened their eyes to the possibilities of careers in the Community Dental Service. He also had instigated a course for the new Diploma in Dental Public Health at Bristol. The diploma had been established by the Royal College of Surgeons as a postgraduate qualification tailored to the needs of the Community Dental Service and improve its career structure. Almost all Avon Community Dental Officers appointed after this time had sessions in the Dental School which improved the coordination of childrens' dental services in the District, enhanced training, and eased clinical pressures on academic staff.

This was a period of considerable progress for the Dental School. A new timetable was introduced in January 1972 which swept away the old block system of teaching and allowed integrated longitudinal teaching within the clinical course as far as the building permitted. An integrated human disease course had been running very successfully since 1966 and was now firmly established and enjoyed by students and clinical staff.[101] The " Dental Expo" set up by Professor Declan Anderson organised for post O-level secondary school pupils was bearing fruit. Groups of 50 pupils, most of whom had not considered dentistry as a career, were escorted them round the Expo in pairs lead by enthusiastic dental students. The Expo visited Taunton, Bath, Exeter, and Southampton and, at a time when there was a general shortage of good dental applicants nationally, ensured that Bristol had an increasing number of able students applying for its BDS course. Subsequently the General Dental Council published a multimedia project kit based on Expo entitled "The biology of the mouth".

However, by the mid 1970s there was considerable frustration amongst the non-professorial staff at Bristol. This arose for several reasons. First, despite the work to rule by clinical academics which had taken place in 1970, there were still considerable discrepancies between their terms of employment and those of junior hospital staff of equivalent NHS status. Secondly, in comparison with schools of similar intake (Cardiff,

The London, Kings, UCL and the Royal Dental) Bristol was less well staffed and, based on UGC figures, clearly spent significantly less per capita on its dental students. Finally, Bristol's non-professorial staff felt they had no input into the running of the Dental School. Decisions rested entirely in the hands of the three clinical professors. A typical example of this was the Dental School Library which was run by Professor Darling as his Departmental Library (which technically it still was!). Matters came to a head in May 1974 when he refused to buy any of the five books recommended to him by the Board of Dental Studies Library sub-committee.

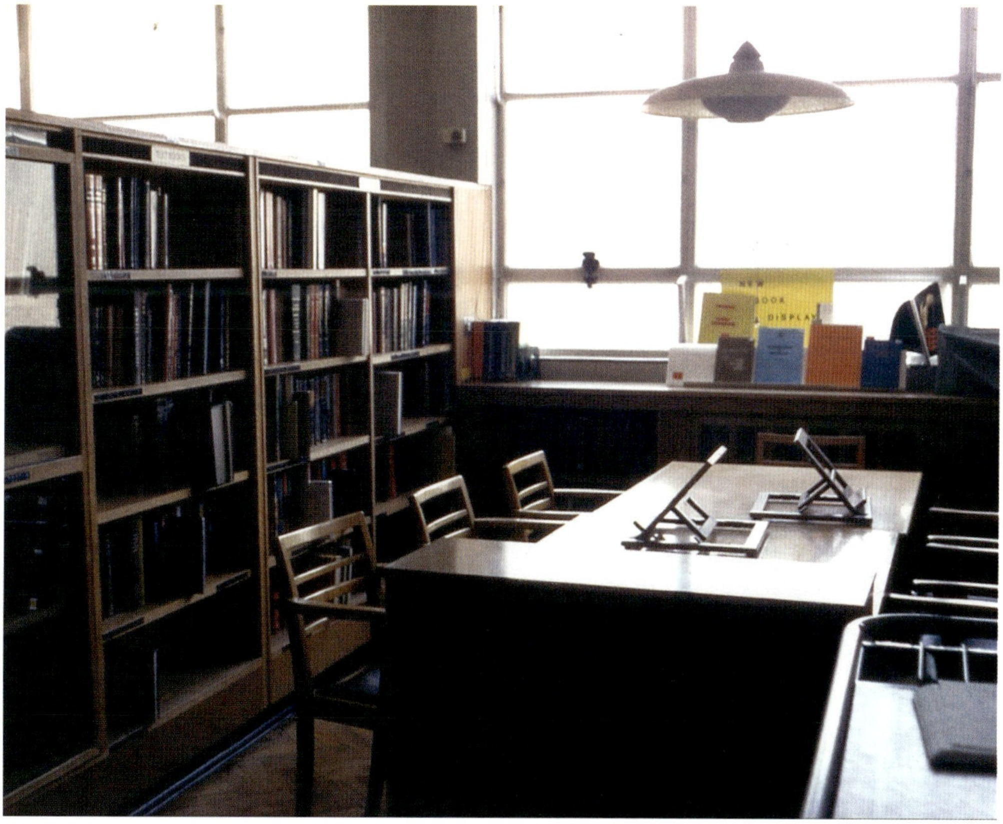

Figure 56. The old Dental Library: its space on the first floor now part of the Child Dental Health clinic.

The Board, ably and courageously led by Graham (later professor) Charlton, insisted at its meeting of that month that the library be taken over by the Medical Library and established on a proper footing. It was after this singular meeting that Professor Darling largely disengaged himself from the running of the School. While in the past there had been edicts following closed meetings of the three clinical professors these almost ceased and the School drifted.[102]

On a happier note on March 19th 1975 a meeting had taken place between Bristol University and members of the UGC to discuss:

"capacity aspects and the overall teaching pattern in connection with further proposals for Dental Hospital and School expansion and also Phase II of the BRI development".[103]

Almost all other UK dental schools had acquired new sites and large new buildings during the preceding decade of generous earmarked funding for dentistry. The University now wanted to press for 60 student places at Bristol and the UGC invited the University to submit proposals for a "first phase of an ultimate project" to take care of the clinical and academic needs of the Dental Hospital and School. There could hardly have been a worse time to try to accomplish such a jointly funded building. Fortunately the site of about one acre on the south side Upper Maudlin Street as far

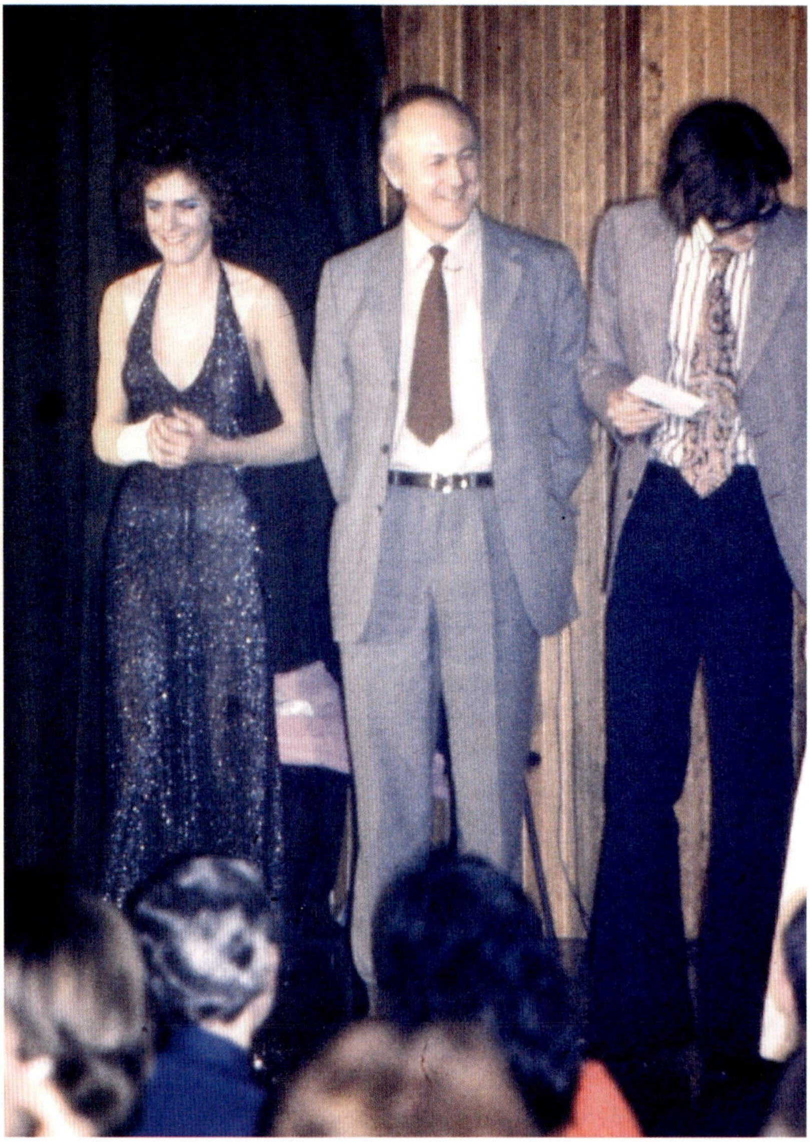

Figure 57 .The popular Graham Charlton at the Dental "Smoker" of 1972.

as Johnny Ball Lane had been acquired by the Special Trustees of the United Bristol Hospitals who correctly saw it as crucial for the development of hospitals on the site. This they now offered to the Regional Health Authority, pointing out that the Dental School had already gained agreement of the University and the University Grants Committee for what would become the 1985 extension to the school.[104] The remainder of the site would eventually become the UBHT Teaching block.

Inflation was now out of control in the UK, it peaked at 25% in 1975, and the Labour Government's efforts to control it were followed by strikes which led to Margaret Thatcher's Conservative victory in the 1979 general election. The new government immediately imposed severe restriction on the finances of universities as well as stringent limitations on the spending of hospital authorities. The following year the justification for public scrutiny of universities finances was provided by Sir Peter Swinnerton Dyer's valedictory address as Vice Chancellor of Cambridge where he drew a picture of sherry swilling dons abandoning teaching and research in middle age and fading away on full pay.[105] The Committee of Vice Chancellors and Principals immediately announced that it was looking into the tenure system with a view to being able to make it easier for academic staff to be made redundant.[106] Hard pressed clinical academic staff greatly resented being tarred with the same brush as Oxbridge dons and the prospect of the loss of tenure only accelerated the movement of able young medical and dental academics into secure and better paid hospital posts and academic jobs overseas. Senior dental staff at Bristol, like those in other schools, felt it was wise to grab promotion wherever it came available rather than hope to achieve it at their own University. So while Arthur Darling had been able to claim in the autumn of 1979 that no fewer than 14 Bristol dental staff had been appointed to chairs in schools in the UK and overseas[107] two of the most recent were to be Bob Yemm (to a Senior Lectureship and later a personal chair in Dundee) and Jim Fletcher (to a chair in Liverpool). These had been regarded by many as heads of department in waiting at Bristol. Other staff to depart at around this time were Graham Charlton to a Chair at Edinburgh and Bill Deubert to head up the new school in Papua New Guinea.

Another great loss shortly afterwards was the untimely death of John Farrell in June 1981. John, as Postgraduate Dental Dean had been a leader in continuing postgraduate education. His courses organised under Section 63 of the NHS Act , known locally in the Region as "Dental Roadshows", were far ahead of their time and by the mid 1970s had achieved a 60% participation among dentists in the South West. His work, coupled with his election to the General Dental Council, was to lead to the acceptance that there should be formal continuing professional development (CPD) requirements for all dental practitioners.[108]

Against a background of increasingly severe university cuts contemporary dental research was revealing that there was a declining prevalence of dental disease in the UK and most industrialised countries which was most marked in children and had implications for dental manpower.[109] To make matters worse, Professor Lehner and his colleagues at Guys were showing from their primate studies that there was reason to believe that a vaccine could be developed against dental caries.[110] Dental academic and NHS staff at Bristol felt particularly insecure. From their perspective they now occupied a small overcrowded school which was vulnerable to any cuts which might be made to the UK dental student intake. Their concerns did not seem to be shared by the three dental professors, perhaps, because these were now looking forward to their retirement! In their frustration the University non-professorial and NHS staff wrote a "round robin" to the Vice Chancellor, Sir Alec Merrison, to ask him to intervene in order to establish a viable management framework for the future of the School. Professor Bob Chambers, the Pro Vice Chancellor responsible for the Faculty of Medicine at the time, was asked to take this on. His report which was undertaken in consultation with the non professorial staff and Heads of other leading UK dental schools appeared in February 1981 and received universal support. Over the next 10 years its recommendations were gradually put into effect and it remained the structural basis of the school until 2008 (See page 145).

Professor Arthur Darling retired in July 1982. Many generations of Bristol Dental students contributed very generously to his retirement gift of £1100 which went towards a lathe for his passion for woodwork. (The two staves he made for the Royal College of Surgeons of England when Vice Dean of the Faculty of Dental Surgery are still in use and are witness to his considerable wood carving skills).There was also a good sum left over for him to purchase tools of his own choice. Arthur was very greatly touched by the gifts, as well as the book containing several hundred signatures. A dinner was organised in his honour. This was the first of two instances when the Vice Chancellor Sir Alec Merrison failed to arrive for an important dental function. Fortunately on this occasion the VC was at home at Stuart House and duly arrived at high speed in his mini to undertake the presentation.

The same month saw work finally beginning on the new extension mooted 7 years earlier. Because it proved impossible to obtain an NHS contribution for a joint building it was finally agreed by the UGC to press ahead with a purely university funded building adjacent to the 1974 Wellcome building.[111] Sadly the fixed sum for what had been planned as a 5 storey building in 1975 had been so eroded by inflation during the late 1970s that in the end only a three story building could be afforded.

Arthur Darling was succeeded in October 1982 by the energetic and uncompromising Professor Crispian Scully. At his appointment the Vice Chancellor Sir Alec Merrison made it clear that they wished him to shake the school in to action and re-establish its high reputation.[112] The first he most certainly did. He soon had a notice on his desk which stated "Have you a problem – or are you the problem?". The name of the old department of Oral Medicine was changed to become "Oral Medicine, Surgery and Pathology" in line with the Chambers Report . Dr David Poole took over as acting head of the MRC Dental Unit while the MRC pondered its future. Earlier that year Professor Declan Anderson, who was by then President of the British Division of the International Association of Dental Research, had written to the dental press to voice his concern that three sets of interviews over 5 years had failed to produce a replacement for Arthur Darling as director of the Unit.

Professor Stephens who had been the University's mute observer on the MRC's latest Search Committee was of the opinion that its members regarded all areas of dental research as being within the capabilities of one person and should really have been solved by now. As their search for a Leonardo progressed, a series of able and internationally recognised research workers were dismissed in turn as " not quite what we are looking for"; "operating in a rather restricted field"; "lacking in breadth of vision we need" etc. This greatly angered the UK dental research community. Their concerns were voiced when Sir James Gowan presented the MRC's 1981/82 annual report in November 1983.[113] However a year later the future of the Unit was still unknown. In the end Professor Newell Johnson, who had trained at Bristol and obtained his PhD at the School in 1968 was appointed. He held this title at the Royal College of Surgeons, London for 10 years jointly with that of Nuffield Professor of Dental Science. The Bristol Unit was allowed to continue to exist as long as its staff were able to fund themselves from project grant money. This they did very successfully for a number of years under the leadership of Dr David Poole who had himself applied for the MRC Unit Directorship in 1983 only to be judged to be not what they were looking for. It is hugely to his credit that this greatly respected member of staff, who was also known to many generations of university students as the very approachable warden of Hiatt Baker Hall, never seemed to show any ill feeling for this lack of recognition.

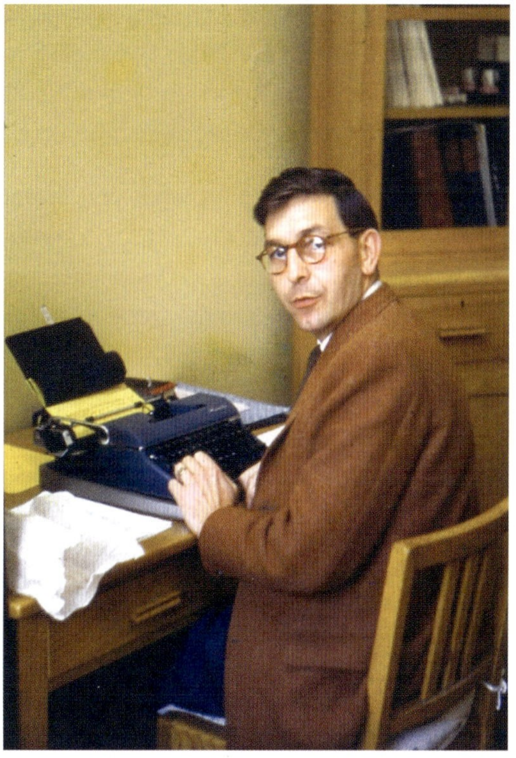

Figure 58. The late Dr David Poole in 1963.

The GDC's visitation to the School in late January 1983 had judged the Bristol course as "sufficient", and one of only four schools seen at that time as having an adequate dental course. However the visitors noted "a certain diffuseness in the administrative structure" of the School and expressed the view that definitive arrangements for its departments should be established as soon as possible. They also expressed the hope that the clinical chairs which were about to become vacant through retirement would be filled immediately though not necessarily in the same disciplines. It should be remembered that up until this time the structure of the Bristol Dental School remained very much that which had been seen in both Britain and America in the 1940s with departments of Dental Medicine, Dental Surgery, and Dental Prosthetics with Orthodontics, the latter two being grouped because of their dependence on dental laboratory support. By this time all other UK dental schools had adopted a structure which recognised the common bases of contemporary dental teaching.

The GDC was only urging what was already in place at other UK schools and also reflecting the Chambers report's recommendations which had been made known to them. The UGC Medical and Dental Subcommittee at its visit on 9th December of the same year also alluded to the same need for reorganisation when Professors Bradford, Berry and Anderson retired. They also observed that clinical medicine and dentistry was 20% under funded by the University whilst preclinical subjects were over funded by a similar amount.[114] The University chose to disagree on the grounds that historically all universities had been subsidising their dental schools and so it continued to use the same funding model for several years to the School's considerable disadvantage.[115]

The new UGC funded school building was finally completed in February 1984 at a cost of £881,427. There was no money for a physical link to the existing buildings on the site but these were added later with NHS funds. Because significant cost cutting had taken place the ground floor remained as an "undercroft" . It served initially as a covered area for bicycles. The much needed additional clinical space which was originally envisaged in 1975 as a jointly funded UGC/ NHS building took a further 10 years to achieve. Nevertheless the increased office, laboratory and library space had a very beneficial effect on staff morale and the "temporary" staff accommodation which had been rented for 10 years in Manulife House was finally relinquished in 1988.

The formal opening of the building took place on Saturday 24th March 1984. The many alumni and guests expected to see the Vice Chancellor unveil a plaque to mark this significant development. For reasons which were not entirely clear at the time, Sir Alec Merrison failed to materialise to perform this duty and Professor Bradford ably deputised in his absence. The photograph which subsequently appeared in the University newsletter[116] and various dental journals had to be staged the following week (Figure 60).

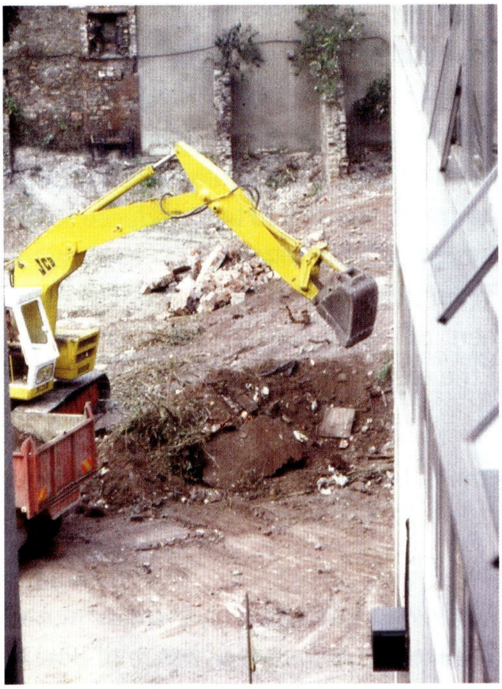

Figure 59. (a) Work starts on the 1984 extension.

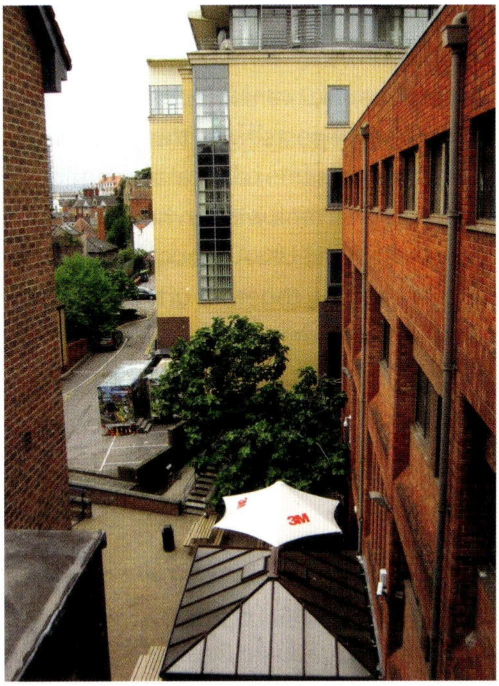

(b) The building as it is today.

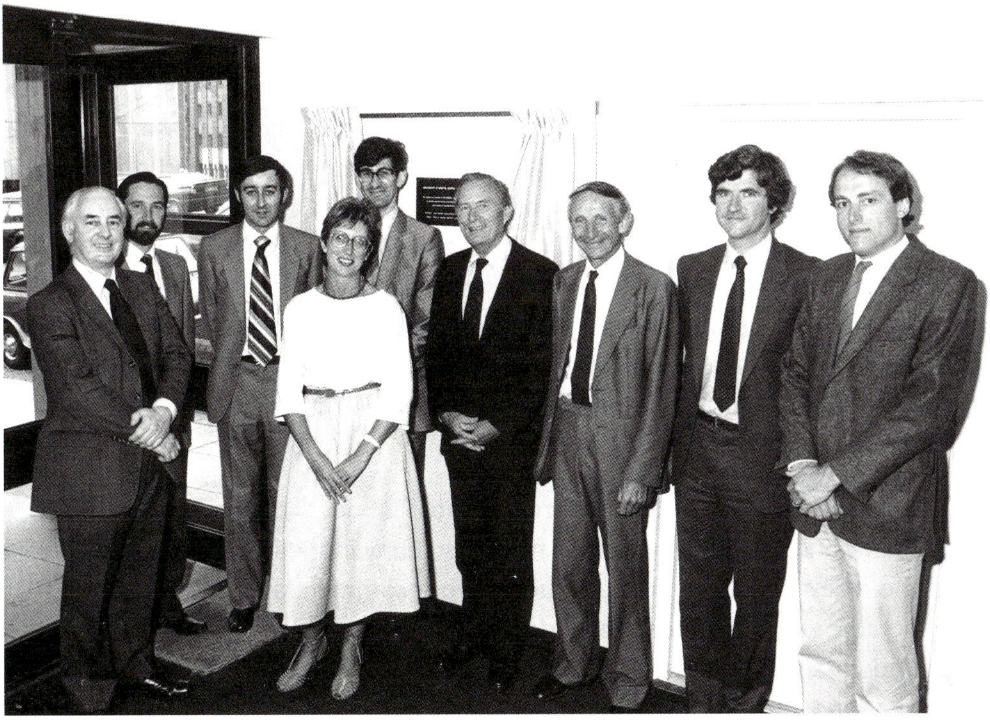

Figure 60. The staged photograph organised after the formal opening of the 1984 Extension to the School.

the University had eased somewhat and the School was given permission to fill the chair shortly to be made vacant by Professor Bradford's retirement. It was agreed that this would be in the field of restorative dentistry and that the appointee would then take over as head of a new Department of Restorative Dentistry which would combine what had been the separate departments of conservation and dental prosthetics. The front runners for appointment were to be Richard Elderton (Dundee) and Alan Harrison (Leeds). In the end Richard Elderton, with a background in conservative dentistry was appointed. His research work started while he was at Dundee was very topical, if unpopular among NHS general dentists, for it had shown that replacement of existing restorations invariably resulted in further loss of tooth substance and weakening of the tooth. It indicated that, wherever possible, a preventive approach followed by a period of observation should be undertaken.[126] At the time this was being proposed, Professor Roger Anderson and his colleagues at Birmingham were reporting on the decline in caries, especially amongst children[127] and some voices in the dental press and BDA's Dental Manpower sub Committee were soon expressing concern that there might be future unemployment in the dental profession.

The names of two former Bristol dental graduates appeared in the 1986 New Year Honours list. Mike Treweeke for many years a Recognised Teacher in Dental Surgery as well as our Lecturer in Dental Jurisprudence received the MBE and Harry Orton, Consultant Orthodontist at Kingston General Hospital the OBE.

Professor Eric Bradford, retired in great style at a party held on 6th June 1986.This started in the Students Common Room before proceeding to a formal dinner and presentation. One of the first things he did in his retirement was to institute the presentation of a Student President Tankard the first recipient being Rod Ferguson the recently qualified 1984 Student President.

By this time the Old Student Common Room was being converted into an enlarged Primary Care Unit and Consultant suite. No firm plans for a new student common room had yet appeared. The title of the student revue of 1984 "Last Orchards at the Bar" records the discovery made by the diligent Unit Administrator, that the old student common room had been operating for some years without a bar licence!

Kathy Orchard the Dental unit administrator, whose husband was a senior manager with Whitbread, soon realised that the student common room's previous licensing arrangements were illegal. To her huge credit, Kathy with the Student Senior President, Iain Hathorn and a number of key undergraduates, including Jon Moore and Martin Fulford, pushed for a new common room, which would have a properly licensed bar.

Eric Bradford was to return on October 25th 1986, to attend the celebrations surrounding the opening of the new Student Common and Bar which were sited

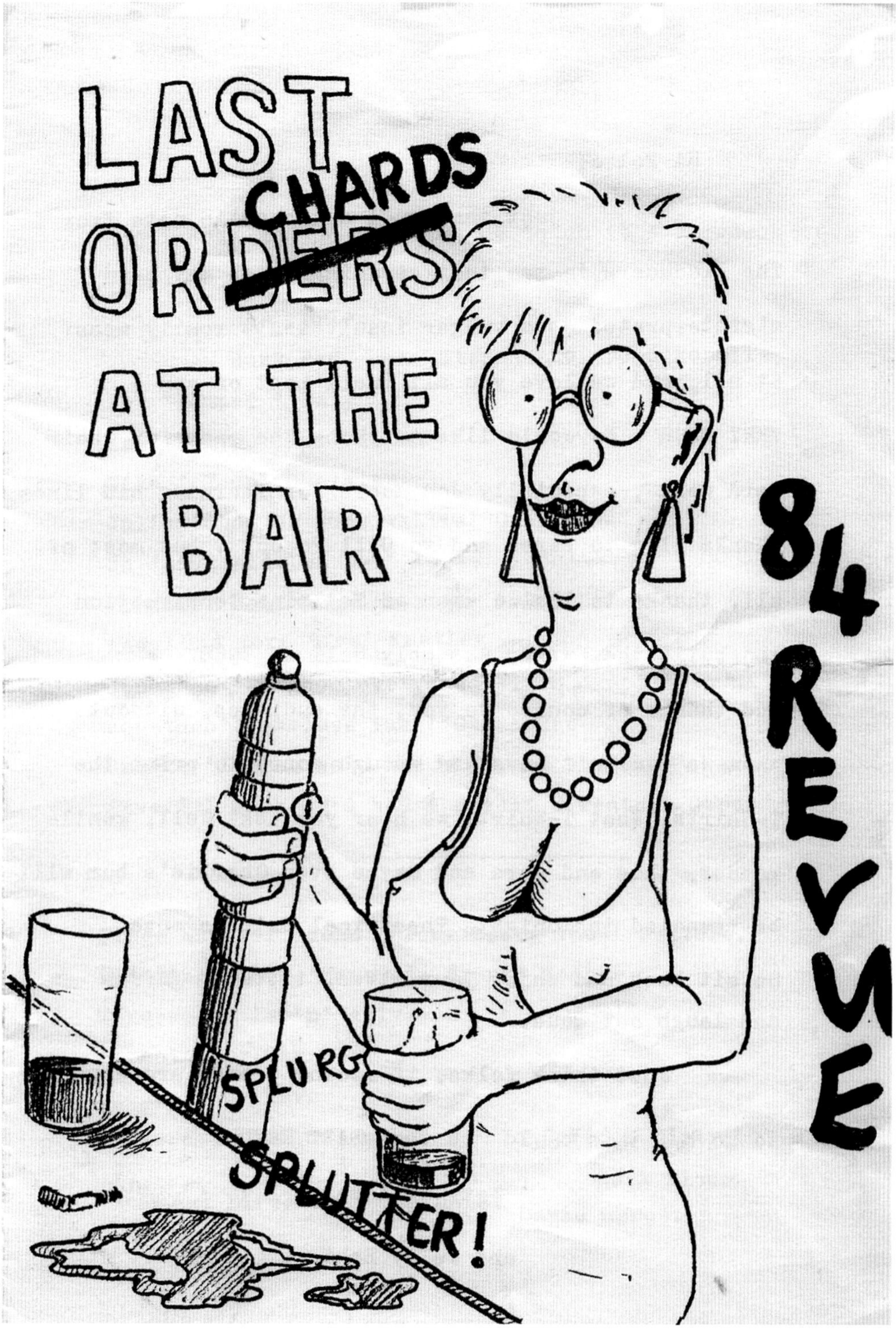

Figure 61. The programme for the Student Review of 1984.

in the undercroft of the 1985 extension. In review of available space some months before it had been deemed, unfit for model and equipment storage, but suitable for dental students! The funding for the conversion to a student common room and bar was achieved through sizeable contributions from the Special Trustees of the United Bristol Hospitals and the Bristol and Weston Health Authority.[128] Further money, for the internal furnishings was raised through the efforts of the student committee, with donations from the Bristol Dental Alumni Association, dental supply companies and dental defence organisations.

The bar required a licence, which was arranged through the local magistrate's court. The first licensee was Iain Hathorn. On attending the court, the Dental Hospital licensee was to be considered alongside a request from the Bishop of Bristol. Owing to the need, for the said licensee, to get back to treat his patients, the magistrate considered the Dental Hospital license ahead of the Bishop!

The Bristol Dental School licence is the only one which now exists in a UK Dental School. The bar opened every Friday night and was a great opportunity for staff and students to meet together and let off steam, as required, at the end of a busy week. It also allowed several special events / parties to take place legally. It has run very well over the twenty and more years it has existed and remains solvent, although the bar finances have been a matter of mystery. The bar managers have the life-long honour of free booze, when in town. The opening hours and the nature of the license remain largely unchanged. In 2009, the old bar in the undercroft was moved to premises very close by and retains its name, "The Hathorn Bar".

By this time national changes were afoot. The Royal Dental Hospital School of Dentistry had merged with Guy's Hospital Dental School in 1983 and the BDA Manpower subcommittee was now recommending a further 10% cut in the dental intake nationally.[129] In the light of this the University Grants Committee set up a Working Party chaired by Professor Moore of Manchester to make recommendations regarding the future of dental education in the UK. All dental schools were visited between February and October 1987, Bristol received its visitors on 29th September l987 only six weeks after Professor Harrison took up his appointment when the funding for Professor Berry's frozen chair was finally released. Alan thus held the unique honour of having undergone this revue exercise twice in both Leeds and Bristol dental schools. Given the tremendous effort which the school had put in since Crispian Scully's arrival he and we were quietly confident.

In October 1987 Arthur Darling was again seen in the School and exchanged a few words with many former colleagues, enquiring with interest as to how the School was surviving. He looked just the same and asked after everyone in a friendly way. It was only when we heard of his death just before Christmas that we realised this had been his farewell to the School.[130] By this time the arrangements for an oil painting of Arthur had already been agreed funded from contributions from the Bristol Dental Alumni and many individual past students and members of staff .It meant that this was ready to be unveiled in May 1989 in the presence of Mrs Darling and members of the University, School and Health Authority.

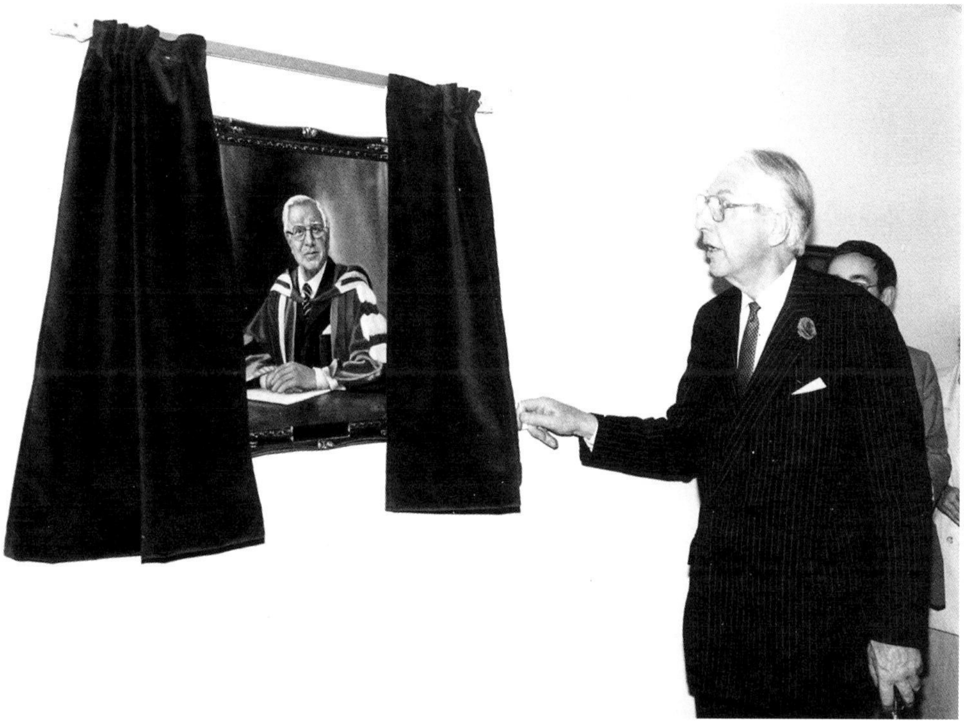

Figure 62. Charles Clarke, former Chairman of the Bristol and Weston Health Authority, unveiling the portrait of Professor Darling which now hangs in the Dental School.

When the results of the UGC Dental Working Party had been announced in February 1988 they contained the proposal that the University of Dundee Dental School and the University College Dental School should close, Guy's Hospital Dental School was to reduce its dental student intake but Cardiff and Leeds were to increase theirs. As had been the case with the earlier UGC research assessment exercise the basis for such decisions was unclear. To quote Naylor (1989):

"An especially sinister and thoroughly divisive aspect of the Report was the grading of the Schools into category ratings.. A being excellent B -average and C - Below Average The rating of the school was not contained in the Terms of Reference nor was it mentioned before or during the inquiry. Further at no stage since the report was published has adequate reason been offered to justify this inclusion."[131]

Bristol was graded as C (below average) but much more damaging was the content of the Report, which stated that the Committee's first inclination had been to recommended Bristol for closure and that it was only the case made by the Regional Health Authority, that without the Dental Hospital and School it would be impossible to deliver effective specialist dental services to the South West Region which saved us. The shock and disbelief at Bristol was shared by staff at Dundee Dental School who could not see on what basis they had been chosen for closure in preference to Edinburgh. In a superbly researched and argued case, which appeared in late 1988, the Dundee School was able to prove that on all the criteria that the Report might have used, far from being the least effective school Dundee was in fact the most effective in the UK. The UGC then reversed their decision and Edinburgh closed.

The Dundee case which examined all UK schools also showed that Bristol came a close second in effectiveness! Their report was forwarded by the Dental School Heads of Department to the Vice Chancellor and the District Health Authority in January 1989. As the Chief Executive of the District Health Authority said at the time "If in the present circumstances you had claimed that Bristol was an excellent dental school I would not have believed you, but when Dundee states it I feel it is very likely to be true". Sadly by this time the damage had been done and for the next thirteen years the new Vice Chancellor Sir John Kingman seemed to be of the view that the University was harbouring a third rate dental school.

Yet another UGC visit took place at the end of May to look at the University generally. These visitors reiterated that 20% of the money which the UGC allocated clinical medicine and dentistry was not in fact passed on to those cost centres whereas preclinical medicine and dentistry received about 20% more that the UGC calculated they should do. The University's response was that, as in a previous visit, they disputed the UGC's findings!

Gloom at this time was not confined to either the Dental School or Bristol University but affected the whole of UK tertiary education. The press was full of accounts of unfilled and frozen academic posts, many of these caused by those who had left for more congenial appointments abroad. As Professor Peter Hall an eminent geographer who had recently emigrated to California said

> *"British Universities are utterly depressing places. To climb out of the gloom and doom everyone is being forced to adopt money grabbing measures."* [132]

In April the Under Secretary of State Robert Jackson announced at the Conference of University Convocations that as part of the Government's strategy to give greater purchasing power to students there would be doubling of University fees to £1200 to encourage "expansion". He also confirmed the Government's plan to split teaching and research funding. The editorial of the Times Higher Education Supplement of the following week summarised the dangers of such a strategy.[133]

For dentistry this was to mark the departure from the Robbins Committee philosophy, which may be paraphrased as "university teaching in an environment of research" which had been followed since the late 1960s.[134] Up until this point dental academics had been free to pursue their research interests in an amateur way rather as an 18th century gentleman might have done. Things were now to become much more professional and competitive. To compete an academic would either have to become a full time research worker or be a member of a group focussed on a particular research problem. While schools such as Guys had sufficient numbers of staff to free some from teaching duties in order to lead grant funded research teams the Bristol Dental School had little possibility of doing so.

When Jon Shepherd (now Professor Jon Shepherd CBE) resigned his post in March 1989 to take up his chair in Cardiff, Professor Scully as Head of School wrote to the Dean of Faculty. He pointed out that with only 22 full time equivalent staff we could not hope to compete with schools of similar student intakes, such as the London Hospital Dental School, with its 60 UGC funded staff. However the view prevailed at the University that the dental school at Bristol was not understaffed, rather that every other UK school was overstaffed!

As further staff departed and posts remained unfilled the School briefly was reduced to 20 FTE posts. Lecturers who were required to undertake 5 clinical teaching / treatment sessions in the terms of their honorary NHS contracts found themselves undertaking 9 clinical sessions. Lectures, letters, administration and exam marking took more than the remaining contractual time and there was no time for research. Stress and depression were all pervading.

In 1989 the UGC undertook a second more comprehensive Research Selectivity Exercise based on "informed peer review" . There were 70 subject review panels, of which clinical dentistry was one. The research output of each school was judged on the basis of submitted evidence and graded as follows:

UGC Research Selectivity Exercise Rating Scheme

1. National level of excellence in none, or virtually none, of the sub-areas of activity.
2. National level of excellence in up to half of the sub-areas of activity.
3. National level of excellence in the majority of the sub-areas of activity; or to international level in some.
4. National level of excellence in virtually all sub-areas of activity; possibly showing some evidence of international excellence; or to international level in some and at

least national level in a majority.

5. International level of excellence in some sub-areas of activity; and national level; in virtually all others.

The School was quietly confident. In a letter to Professor Harrison, his successor as Head of School Professor Scully who had done so much to galvanise research activity in the School, stated:

> *" We have come successfully through the UGC review and I am entirely confident that the Research Selectivity Exercise will prove beyond doubt the radical improvement over that which we have inherited."*[135]

The results were announced in August 1989, some weeks after the UGC had been replaced by the Universities Funding Council (UFC). Bristol University had achieved 5 subject areas rated as 5 and none assessed as 1. Dentistry was rated as 3 as were the majority of the other UK dental schools. We considered ourselves very lucky and knew it was only the three recent professorial appointees who had brought with them their excellent research profiles which had enabled us to achieve a 3. However given the current staffing of the school these new members of staff would find it very difficult to maintain this level of research activity for the next review due in 1992. Sadly as far as the University was concerned we had performed rather poorly but we were relieved to find this rating would have minimal effect on the UFC funding of our dental cost centre for the next three years. But the writing was on the wall: the research component of government funding would soon be dependant on our research grading.

For 5 years the School had been arguing that its university staffing should be brought up to the level which the University Grants Committee was providing for dental teaching and which they and we maintained was the minimum number for a viable dental school. The lack of 5 or 6 core posts was now having very serious consequences for research in the school. Moreover in future any failure to deliver in this area would now impact on funding provided by the UFC for the Dental School.

In April 1989 the four heads of department once again sought the advice of Professor Chambers, author of the 1991 "Chambers Report" on the future structure of the Dental School, who by this time was Chairman of the University's Finance Committee.[136] Professor Chambers was soon convinced of our case and made approaches on our behalf but was overruled. A few months later he was replaced on the Finance Committee. Despite this, at a further meeting with the Dean of Faculty in May 1989 it last appeared to be accepted at Faculty level that the Dental School was under funded but we were also told that because of the current financial climate there was no way that we were going to get any more money in the near future.

So ended the academic year of 1989 which was to be a low point in the history of the Dental School. It was only with the considerable support of our NHS and Community dental staff, who undertook more and more of the undergraduate teaching, and by the prodigious efforts on the part of all University dental staff that were able to claw our way out of a near impossible situation during the next 10 years.

CHAPTER 9

THE LONG ROAD BACK 1990-1999

The table below was the basis of a letter from the Heads of Departments to the Vice Chancellor Sir John Kingman at the end of 1988. In this they identified urgently needed posts which would have brought the staffing of the school to the level of those UK schools of equivalent size in terms of student intake. Nothing was achieved by the meeting and the level of staffing was still the same three years later.

School (No. of students)	Oral Medicine			Oral Pathology			Oral Microbiology			Oral Surgery			Dental Radiology			Periodontology Preventive			Restorative			Prosthetics/ Elderly			Paedodontics			Orthodontics			Total
	P	SL	L	P	SL	L	P	SL	L	P	SL	L	P	SL	L	P	SL	L	P	SL	L	P	SL	L	P	SL	L	P	SL	L	
BRISTOL (50)	1	2	½		1						½						1	½	1	1	3½	1		2		1	1	1		1	19
BIRMINGHAM (80)			1	1	1	6				1	1	3				1	2	4	1	3	6	1	1	3		1	2	1		1	41
CARDIFF (50)		1	1			1				1	1	1				1	1	1	1	2	3	1	2	2			3	1	2		26
DUNDEE (45)	1	1	1								1	2					1	2	1	1	4	1	1	3		½	1		½	1	23
EDINBURGH (45)		2	1	1	1	1				1	1	2			1		1	1	1	3	3	1	2	2	1	2	1		1	2	32
GLASGOW (75)	1	1	1		2	2				1	1	2			½	1	2	2	1	4	2½	1	2	2		2	2	1	2	2	38
LEEDS (60)			1		1	2				1	1	3					2	1	1	2	5	1	1	3	1	1	3		1	3	34
LIVERPOOL (60)	1	2	1		2						1½	2			½	1	2	1½			2½	1	1	3	1	1	2		1	2	29
MANCHESTER (65)		1	1	1	1	1				1	2	4			½		2	1	1	1	4½	1	4	3	1	2	2	1		2	38
NEWCASTLE (75)				1	1	2					3	2			1		1	2	1	2	6	1	1	4	1	1	1		1	1	33
SHEFFIELD (50)				1	1	2				1	1	3					1	1	1	1	4	1	1	3	1		1		1	1	26
THE LONDON (56)	1	1	1	1		1		1		1	1	1½					1½	1	1	2	1	1	4	3		1	1	1		1	28
KINGS (48)				1	1	2		1	1	1	1	1	1		1		1	2		3	2	1	3	2		2	1		2	2	32
UMDS (88)		1	1		1					1	1	1			1	2	2	1	2	4	3	1	4	3		2	½	1	2	½	35
UCH (50)							1	1		½	1	1				1	3		1	3	4	½	2		1	1		1	1		23

P - Professor SL - Reader/Senior Lecturer L - Lecturer

rwm/29/8/88

Figure 63. A comparison of full time UGC funded staffing UK dental schools in 1988.

In fact there was little the VC could do at this time. However Sir John had written to the Regional Health Authority Chairman, after the meeting in October 1989, urging that the Regional Health Authority fulfilled its obligation to fund additional space for the Dental School and Hospital to match that which had been provided by the UGC in 1985 .There was good sense behind an approach at this time since the NHS was less savagely hit by public sector cuts at this time. Further, as matters stood, even if the School did eventually acquire the additional posts which the UGC felt it needed to be " viable" there was no way in which they could be accommodated without additional space!

In July 1990 Crispian Scully completed his term as Head of School and looked back with considerable satisfaction on what had been achieved during this time.[137] He also noted the paradox...

> "that those who should give support locally *(to the success of the School evident to the world outside)* seemed unwilling to recognise this success or the fact that we are one of the few (cost) centres to have kept their budget in credit".

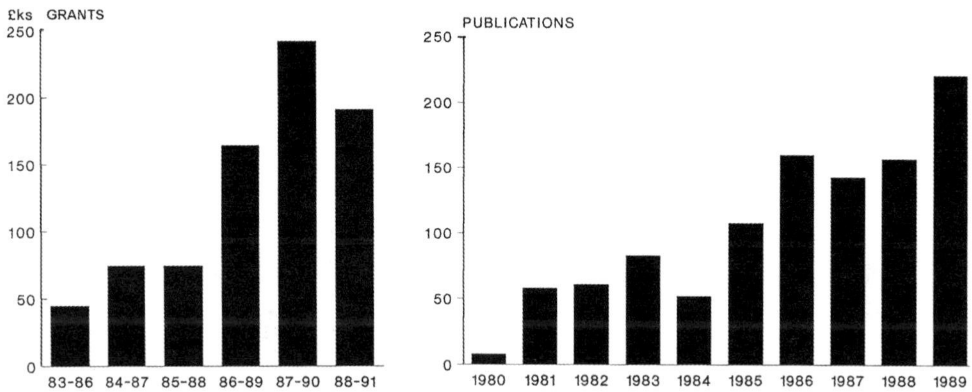

Figure 64. The improving research output of the school in the 1980s as shown by grants and publications.

A further reorganisation of the NHS received the Royal Assent in August 1990. This was not before a group of hospital consultants, lead by Professor Keen of Guys, had unsuccessfully taken the Government to the High Court for authorising expenditure to implement the NHS and Community Care bill before it had received the Royal assent! In the changes which the Act brought about the Dental School lost its representative on the District Health Authority.[138] Nevertheless the previous three years had enabled a number of links to be established which would continue to help us in the coming years . At this time we were held in high regard by the DHA for our ability to run within budget. Indeed, well they might for the old District Health Authority, having clawed itself back into balance from a £1.5 million overspend was now told to make further cuts. The £40,000 planned under spend which the Dental School had been expecting to roll forward for capital works disappeared into this new black hole!

The first Dental Alumni Newsletter appeared in the year 1991 when Dr Reg Andlaw took on the dual roles of Alumni Chairman and Newsletter Editor. The first issue of just 9 pages rapidly swelled under his editorship to a regular 30 pages. Ten years later Reg was asking whether "Newsletter "was still an appropriate title, however such it has remained now for 20 years. By this time it had been agreed nationally to implement the Dental Strategy Review Group's recommendation that the dental course be increased to 5 years. All UK schools were disappointed to find that the additional funding was only to be provided at the preclinical level. Since the whole rationale had been to decongest the clinical course this seemed extraordinary. There was also the problem of how this change could be managed since the only way such an increase could be implemented was for there to be no preclinical student entry in October 1991. Fortunately the UFC agreed there would be level funding for the years of reduced student numbers (1991/2 - 1993/4) to enable these changes to take place.

The Dental Hospital had by now become the Dental Directorate of the new United Bristol Healthcare Trust one of the "first wave" of Trusts in the latest reorganisation of the NHS which was relatively protected during a time of public expenditure cuts. The new Directorate combined the Community and Hospital Dental Services and the planned contraction of the former released capital for the planned refurbishment of many of the clinical areas on the second floor during this period when there were temporarily reduced clinical student numbers.

The new clinical Department of Child Dental Health, relocating orthodontics and paediatric dentistry in what had been the old Histopathology Laboratory, was completed during 1990/1991. The teaching of histopathology by this time was using data projection rather than employing 50 sets of histology slides examined by students using microscopes. Child Dental Health became the only clinical department to be opened twice, the second occasion being opportunistic when on 3rd March 1991 the local MP and Minister of Health the Rt. Hon. William Waldegrave was due to open the "Abbot's

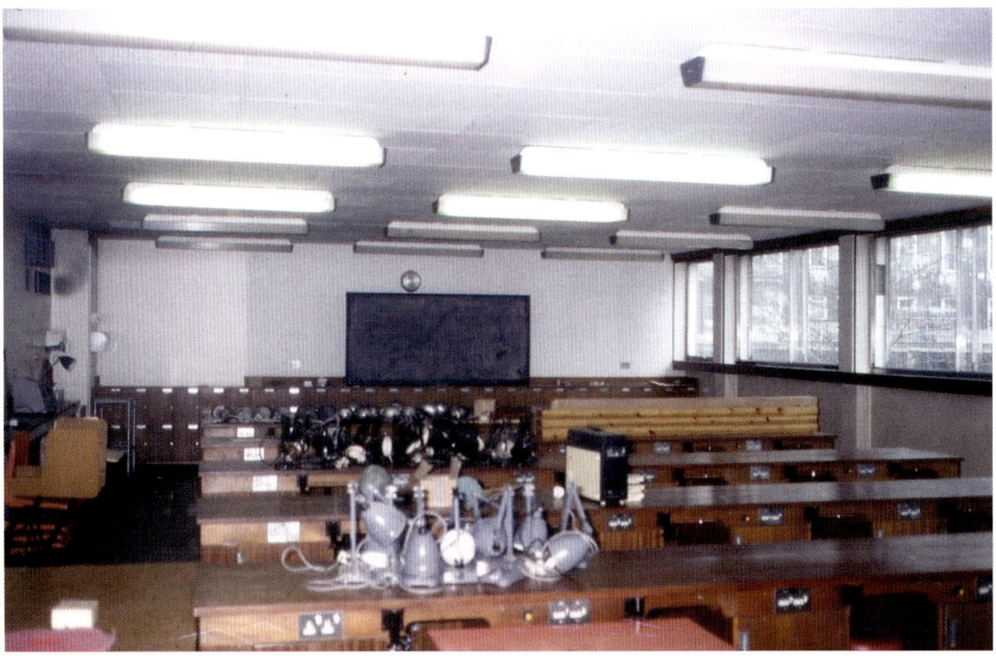

Figure 65 (a) The old histopathology lab on the second floor was replaced in 1991 by the new...

House" for the Special Trustees of the United Bristol Hospitals. The Minister's inspection of the School and new department that day gave an opportunity to emphasise to him the need which the School now had for NHS investment to match the funding of the UGC 1985 building – i.e. to build what would become the Chapter House. The Trust finally agreed to this in 1992. In the same year, the rolling programme for re-equipping conservation (Adult Dental Health) was completed having been temporarily decanted into the new Child Dental Health area.

Financially these were still difficult times for the University which by November 1990, despite its best efforts, had a £4M deficit. The Medical Research Council found itself with a rising £2.5M deficit. As a result all government funded medical research was cancelled until the end of the financial year. Then on the 28th November Mrs Thatcher resigned as Prime Minister and John Major took over as leader of the Conservative Party.

Despite the very unfavourable financial climate the policy of the Government was for university expansion while at the same time expecting the maintenance of high quality research. As the Vice Chancellor was to say in his address to Court on 10th Jan 1991:

> *"The fundamental problem remains, and maybe summed up in the single word investment...This requires investment at all levels, and that investment requires political decision either to commit public funds or to call on private sources. Our politicians, unlike those of our competitor countries, will not invest until prosperity has been achieved. They want the impossible, profit first and investment last."*[139]

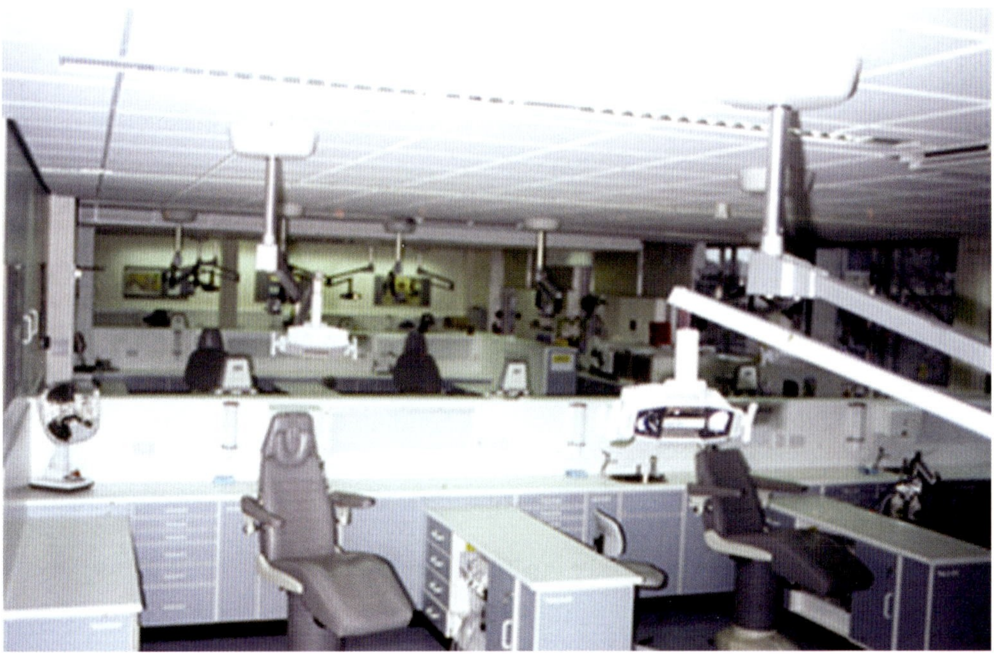

Figure 65 (b) ...Child Dental Health department before becoming part of an enlarged Adult Dental Health clinic in 2009

The Dental School had been increasing the number of postgraduates as fast as it could in order to preserve the funding it received from the University. A sizeable proportion were from overseas although this number received a set back during the first Gulf War. From 4 postgraduates in 1982 there were 19 in 1987. This figure would rise to 30 by 1995. Despite this extra effort the School was required to make a 15% saving on University revenue expenditure in that academic year. Fortunately Professor Harrison, now Head of School, had developed a staffing plan on the sound advice from Sue Delve of the Finance Department which included the funding of a wish list of new staff including a departmental manager who would be needed if the school became a single department with a unified budget. It was possible to achieve the savings without any staff losses by agreeing that none of these new posts would be filled.

At about this time the basement of the School came under scrutiny and was deemed to be a fire hazard. Admittedly housing the inflammable store next to the refectory had not been a very clever idea. While the refectory would eventually be located in the 1995 Chapter House the immediate solution was to use the Eye Hospital refectory which became very crowded. There was also the major problem of how to deal with the 5000 sets of orthodontic models (were these really a fire hazard?). Fortunately it was discovered that there were two huge empty water tanks on the roof of the 1964 extension. These had been installed because earlier planning regulations had required that the Hospital had a full days supply of water stored on site so that it could continue to operate if the public supply was interrupted. Following the first outbreak of Legionnaires Disease in 1977 the decision was taken to bypass such storage. It was now realised that these empty tanks could be removed to release space which, while unfit for human habitation, provided valuable storage space. Since it could only be accessed via an external fire escape an internal model box lift was installed as part of the refurbishment of the second floor.

The year of 1992 was another year of great change. Locally, in anticipation of the 5 year dental course a new curriculum was being slowly introduced. In March we learnt that the supposed 8.5% increase of UFC funding actually mean the University would be £1m worse off in 1992/3![140] In April Peter Ward Booth was appointed as the first Professor of Oral Surgery. This brought the School's academic staffing up to 26 FTEs, the minimum number which the Universities Funding Council had demanded for a viable dental school at Bristol and which they considered they were funding. In fact 5 of these posts were supported by our postgraduate fees.

With an acute shortage of office and postgraduate space, and still no prospect of any major new building, various other possibilities were explored which might be funded by judicious management of the dental equipment revenue budget. The only one of the schemes to come to fruition was an additional floor built on the roof of the

Conversation Department. Because of loading limits placed by the architects this had to be restricted to offices, including those for the newly appointed Professor of Oral Surgery.

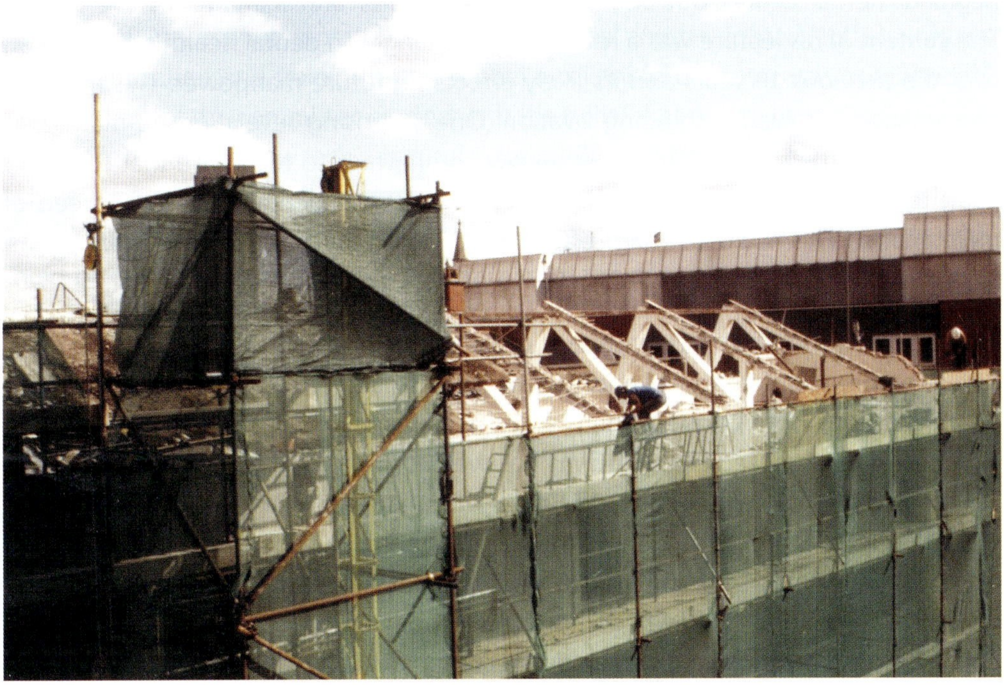

Figure 66. The conservation roof extension offices under construction in March 1992.

By this time, the drift of general dental practitioners away from NHS treatment meant that there was now a shortage of NHS dentists in the UK. This had become acute in the South East, a problem which was highlighted in a leading article in The Times.[141] Matters were made worse when in July 1992, following a retrospective reduction in NHS fees. Both the British Dental Association and the General Dental Practitioners Association voted by an overwhelming majority to accept no more adult NHS patients. Nor were things more peaceful in the Hospital Service where the EEC directives on specialist training and the perceived failure of the UK to implement these appropriately came to a head. The" new deal" on junior hospital doctors hours in 1991 lead quickly to the publication of the Calman Report of 1993[142]. This was to have far reaching effects on the dental as well as medical specialities.

The results of the 1992 Research Assessment Exercise were much as expected and once again showed the high correlation between a UK dental school' s staffing and its research performance .The Bristol Dental School once again boxed above its weight and achieved a three[143] with Oral Medicine and Orthodontics identified as areas of strength. Clinical medicine only managed a grading of two.

dental school. Child Dental Health also saw the departure of Ian Ball to the Community Dental Service .He was replaced by Karen Duncan as Lecturer in Paediatric Dentistry.

Derek Seel was appointed as Postgraduate Dean in 1987 on the retirement of Professor Berry and became responsible for Vocational Training in the Region. Derek was soon to become Dean of the Faculty of Dental Surgery of the Royal College of Surgeons of England and was instrumental in the setting up of its Faculty of General Dental Practitioners in 1992 . He was thus in an ideal position, both nationally and locally to manage the changes in postgraduate dental education which were about to take place. Vocational training, which had been agreed as desirable by a joint BDA, DHS and GDC working party in 1983,[148] became obligatory in 1993 for all newly qualified dentists who wished to become principals in general dental practice within the NHS (It corresponds to what is now known as Dental Foundation Training Year 1).

Derek had established BUOLD (Bristol University Open Learning in Dentistry) in 1990. Based on the Open University this continues to offer over 10 different units of study each year from business skills to dental prosthetics. Each unit involves home study and usually includes 3 study days per year. Students who satisfactorily complete a unit receive 40 credit points towards the Diploma in Dental Postgraduate Studies The first 16 such awards were made in April 1994, and to date over 800 have been made.

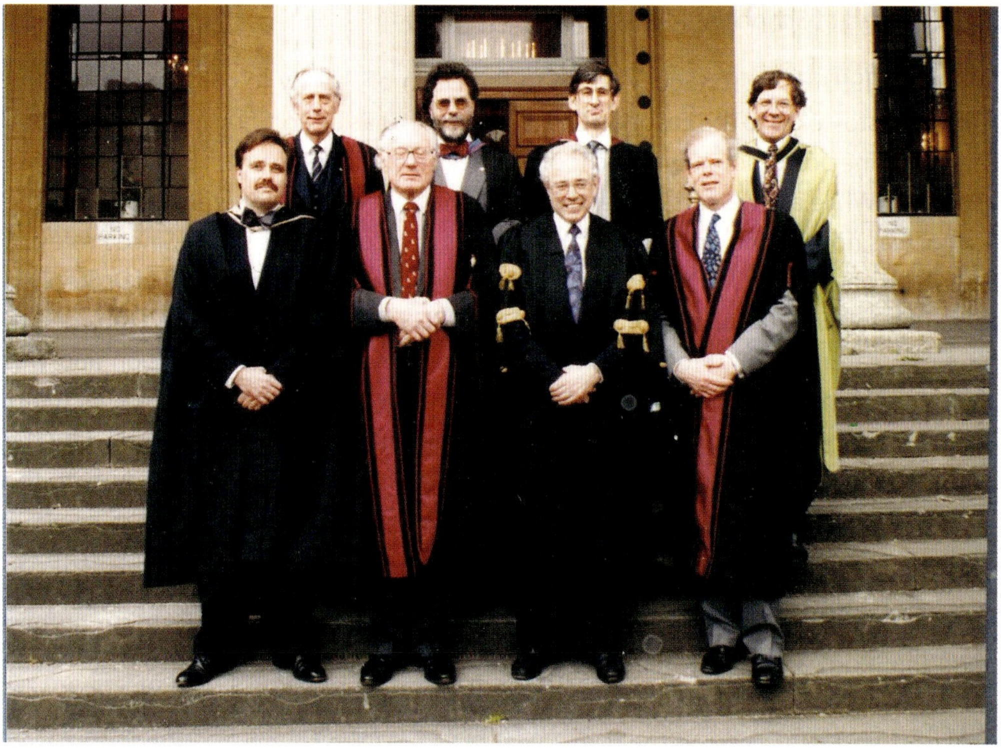

Figure 67. Derek Seel, front row second from left, with some of the BUOLD lead teachers in April 1994.

Early in 1994 the General Dental Council had held a seminar on "The Continuum of Dental Education" and it was clear that continuing professional education would become mandatory in due course. A year later in May 1995 the Chief Dental Officers Report on UK Specialist Dental Training (The Mouatt Report) led to an accord between the Universities, the Dental Faculties of the Royal Colleges of Surgeons, the Postgraduate Dental Deans (COPDEN) and the Specialist Societies which allowed the GDC to progress the introduction of distinctive specialist titles and specialist lists.[149] While their introduction was a logical move, the subsequent requirement that all those who wished to qualify as specialists should undergo a formal College approved training programme caused significant problems for dental schools. Up until that time clinical lecturers who were thought by the University to have progressed to senior lecturer level were assessed by a joint University /Hospital Appointment Committee. Since a senior clinical lecturer appointment carried with it honorary NHS Consultant status there was a an external Royal College Assessor on the committee who had to be convinced of the competence and experience of the candidate. Up until this time this experience was acquired almost exclusively as part of the lecturer's teaching duties. Henceforth formal training was required which included dedicated sessions of supervised personal treatment and attendance on a wide range of specialist clinics. As the lecturer would also have been required to undertake research leading to a higher degree in order to satisfy the University's requirement for promotion to senior lecturer level it meant that the newly appointed lecturer had almost no time to take on undergraduate teaching during his or her first three years. Moreover there was now no point in advertising a vacant lecturers post unless there was the assurance of such training being provided. This did, and still does, cause significant problems for every school.

Shortly after his appointment in September 1993 Dr. Neil Meredith was awarded a prestigious Swedish Research Council Fellowship to continue his implantology research abroad. He left in 1995. While this was a great accolade for the school it caused a major problem in the teaching of conservation. Fortunately matters were helped enormously by the appointment of Paul King as full time NHS Consultant in Conservative Dentistry. He joined Martin Woodhead, Consultant in Dental Prosthetics, who had arrived in 1982. This now meant there were NHS Consultants in all specialty areas of dentistry to support the teaching of junior hospital staff and supervise lecturers on their specialist training programmes.

One of the effects of the need to withdraw lecturers from undergraduate teaching sessions for their own career progression was a reduction in student tutorial time. This was offset by the increasing deployment of home produced computer based teaching. A CAL room which had been established in November 1994 was soon moved to a more appropriate site adjacent to the Dental Library on the first floor of the 1985 extension. The new facility was opened by the Vice Chancellor Sir John Kingman on October 2nd 1995.

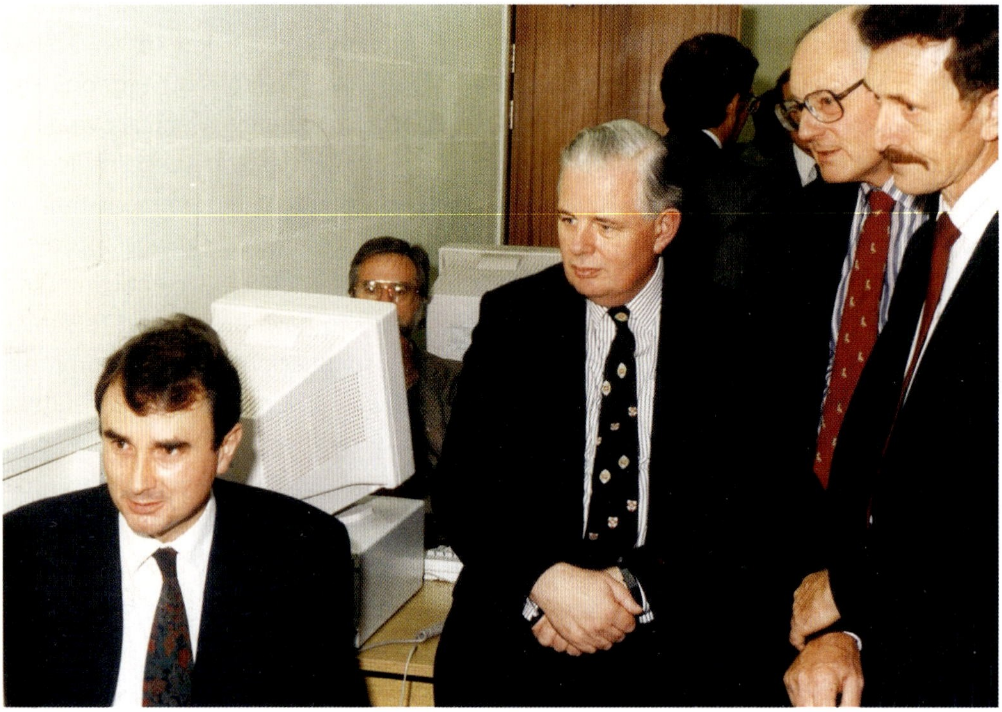

Figure 68. Dr Neil Meredith demonstrates the CAL suite to the Vice Chancellor Sir John Kingman, Derek Seel the Postgraduate Dean and Mr Ken Eaton of the Department of Health.

There had been little progress in the introduction of "professions allied to dentistry" since the publication of the Nuffield Enquiry of October 1993. The Chief Dental Officer Brian Mouatt and the orthodontic speciality[150] were keen to see the introduction of orthodontic auxiliaries to help reduce the long waiting lists for orthodontic treatment which at this time were the cause of more complaints than any other aspect of NHS dentistry. The Standing Dental Advisory Committee's report "Orthodontics in the NHS" had come out strongly in favour of a trial to establish the training requirements for orthodontic auxiliaries. Bristol already had close links with the dental school of the University of British Columbia (UBC) which had been running a highly successful course for Canadian "orthodontic chairsides" for more than 10 years. The difficulty for the UK was that legislation was yet to be put in place to allow those other than dentists to undertake intraoral work. Margaret Seward CBE, who by this time was President of the GDC, was also keen to progress matters. For several years she had been enhancing the training of enrolled dental nurses though the "Teamwork " programme launched in 1991 when she was Editor of the British Dental Journal. In her GDC role she was aware that there were those on the Council who felt that expanded duties nurses, such as the proposed orthodontic auxiliaries, were inappropriate for

NHS dentistry and the Council would not be convinced without the evidence of a UK trial. A plan was therefore devised to invite the UBC team to Bristol to run a trial using dental nurses who had been accepted to train as hygienists just before they commenced their Bristol dental hygiene course. It was argued that as such trainees were permitted to work intraorally they could be viewed starting their course a few days early! "Paper 10" funding was provided by the Chief Dental Officer and the course started in September 1995. Much of this took place in the new hygienists' phantom head room of the Chapter House that had been opened by the Queen and Prince Philip on June 2nd 1995.

However following discussion with Margaret Seward it was agreed that the report of the trial would remain unpublished until the President of the GDC and the Chief Dental Officer decided that the time was right. Under their influence it would then be fast tracked to appear in the British Dental Journal.[151] The paper finally appeared in 1998[152] but not before Professor Stephens had been asked to explain why he had undertaken an illegal and unauthorised trial by the GDC Registrar Norman Davies, much to the embarrassment of its President!

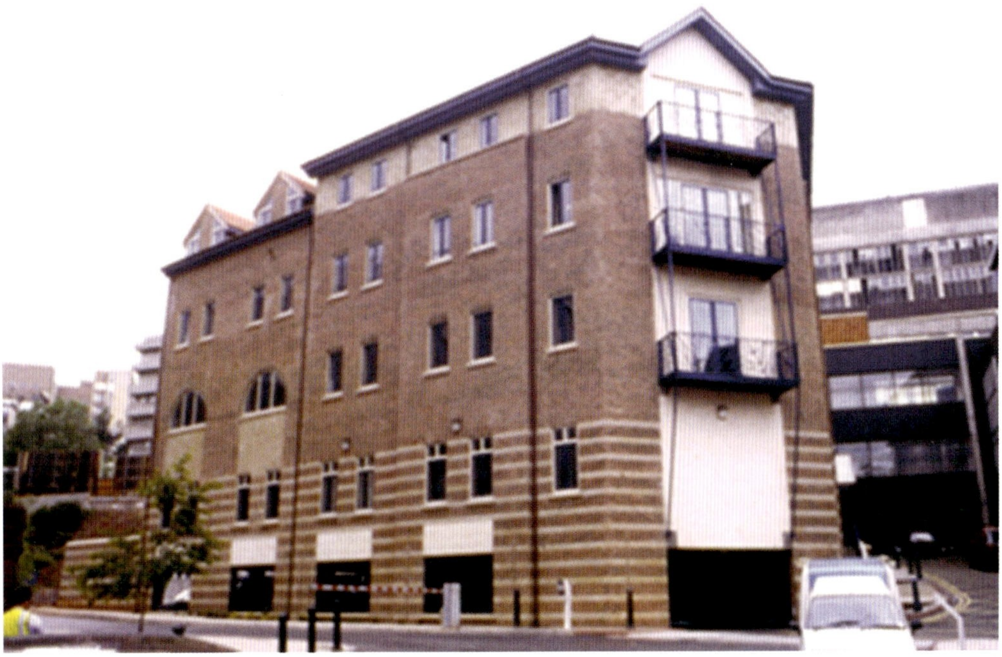

Figure 69. The Chapter House opened in 1995 provided much need teaching and research space.

By now the 1996 UGC Research Assessment Exercise was upon us. The census date for the RAE was 31 March 1996.This was a more serious exercise as there was the intention of research money following research excellence and being removed from those institutions which were seen to perform poorly. There was much discussion as to which staff should be included in the School's submission which would include four examples of their research output. The RAE results, which were published in December, showed the School had improved to a "4" from its grading of 3 in the 1992 Exercise. Once again there was strong correlation between the number of staff in a school and its performance in research. Bristol was again seen to perform better than its staffing would suggest. The School had expected that this result might produce a small increase in funding as the UFC had proposed, but as Clinical Medicine only obtained a grade of 3a, this was diverted by the University to offset their loss of funding.

It had been hoped to refurbish the prosthetic clinic over the summer vacation of 1996 but the lowest tender for the work proved to be well above what the Managers of United Bristol Hospitals Trust had budgeted for. The work was therefore delayed for a year and all the equipment which had been removed in readiness for the upgrading had to be reinstalled. The local press made much of this![153]

Much more serious at this time was the loss of academic staff in medicine and dentistry generally in the UK. This was due to the combined effects of reduced research funding, reduced clinical funding and lack of pay parity with NHS colleagues as Vice Chancellors

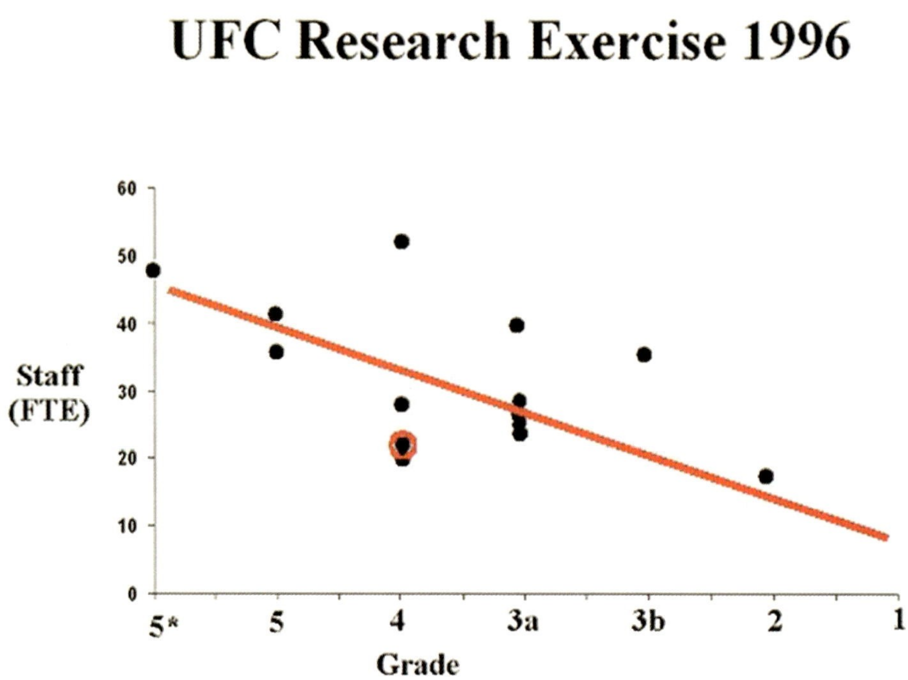

Figure 70. Graph showing the correlation between the number of dental academic staff and performance of UK dental schools to their research grading. Bristol's performance (highlighted) was well above that which might have been expected for a School with only 21 full time equivalent staff.

refused to implement the 1996 Doctors and Dentists Review Body pay award for clinical academics without receiving additional funding from the Government. There were by this time 58 unfilled clinical chairs in medicine and dentistry in the UK.[154] A national enquiry lead by Sir Rex Richardson highlighted what everyone knew: that these posts were no longer attractive.[155] Significantly, the report identified that there were particular problems in dentistry because of the higher level of teaching and service provision undertaken and this ought to receive further attention (para 5.1.7). Needless to say this was never followed up. Finally in December the Government was forced to provide additional money to implement the long overdue pay parity between NHS and Clinical Academic staff .This went some way towards stemming the loss of staff. However at Bristol Professor Elderton resigned in July 1996 to pursue other interests.[156] This led to the creation of a unified Adult Dental Health division under the leadership of Professor Martin Addy comprising conservation, periodontolgy and prosthetics. Professor Alan Harrison was retained as Head of School and Head of the University Department of Oral and Dental Sciences as the School was now known. Alan had recently been appointed Honorary Dental Surgeon to the Queen his after 25 years service in the Territorials. During this time he had been a commander of two major hospitals in the Royal Army Medical Corps (V) which he left with the rank of Colonel.

Fortunately in the same year the School was able to attract Jonathan Cowpe to take up the Chair in Oral Surgery which had been vacant since 1994 following the resignation of Peter Ward Booth. Like so many at this time Peter had decided to accept an NHS consultant post. Jonathan's appointment marked the end of an unsettled period within oral surgery at the school following the departure of the senior lecturer Jon Shepherd for a chair at Cardiff in 1991 and Jack Ross' retirement in 1993. There were also significant changes in the laboratories at this time following the retirements of Terry Foad the Dental Laboratory Superintendent and instructors Graham Biddlecome and Terry Warren.

One of the significant achievements at the end of 1996 was the appointment of Dr Klaus Jandt as Senior Lecturer in Biomedical Engineering and Biomaterial Science. Up until this time dental materials teaching had been undertaken by clinical staff but Klaus's appointment placed teaching on a more satisfactory basis and also made a significant contribution to research. Indeed the patents which he and Dr Robin Mills gained on the application of blue light emitting diodes to the curing of dental composites still benefits the School 10 years later.[157]

In 1997 the General Dental Council published "The first five years - the undergraduate curriculum". This was to be the first of what would become a series of guidelines for the dental undergraduate curriculum.[158] Looking back it seems curious now that up until this time the GDC was content to leave each school to teach as it thought fit rather than follow any nationally agreed guidelines. This was approach was intended to encourage innovation but had disadvantages for the public. For example, it had led to the unwritten decision at Bristol never to shortlist graduates applying for resident house officer posts from one particular school because of their lack of oral surgery experience! The 1997 GDC report also identified undergraduate training as the first phase of lifelong learning. Subsequent research showed that many graduates did not feel they possessed all the skills which their teachers believed they should possess on qualification. Moreover not all of these were acquired during the vocational training year.[159] This was to have a significant effect on dental education in future years and lead to a list of specific learning outcomes in the second GDC report published in 2002. [160]

Roger Smith, Consultant Senior Lecturer in Periodontlogy died in April 1997 after a long fight against cancer.[161] This a was a sad loss of a much respected colleague who, until the arrival of Professor Martin Addy, had been the mainstay of periodontal teaching at the School. Roger first came to Bristol in 1966. He later became responsible for DSA training and was the author of the "The Dental Surgery Assistants Handbook" the highly regarded standard UK text for many years. He is still remembered today in the Roger Smith undergraduate prize.

The New Labour Party, led by Tony Blair, came to power in May 1997. One of the preelection promises had been to "save the NHS". In 1992 Robin Cook had stated that if elected the Labour administration would put £1 billion into NHS dentistry.[162] During Tony Blair's 10 years in office with 40 successive quarters of economic growth, NHS funding greatly increased to 9% of GDP[163] but little found its way into the dental services. So in 1997 while there were nearly 30,000 dentist on the Register, under 17,000 were working in the General Dental Services.

By 1998 the School had 12 undergraduate computers and nearly 60 CAL programmes available for students from 8.00am till 6.00pm. There was a central server logging system to monitor how these were being used. A number of research papers came out of this.[164 165] Not surprisingly Bristol final year students were shown to have far greater IT skills and confidence than those in other UK dental schools.[166] The GDC had published its consultative document on reaccreditation and recertification for the dental profession in 1997[167] with the prospect of proof of CPD hours becoming mandatory in due course. By this time the Department of Health had realised that computer assisted learning, designed for today's undergraduates, was equally effective for updating yesterday's graduates. Selected programmes, including those produced in Bristol were taken up by the Department of Health for this purpose.

The second edition of *The First Five Years – A framework for Dental Undergraduate Education* was published by the General Dental Council in August 2002. As with the first edition the overall intention was to define the scope and content of the undergraduate curriculum. However the second edition included, for the first time, a list of specific learning outcomes. This reflected a sea change in national attitudes towards university education. Up until 1990 universities had been regarded as places where students came to learn rather than places where they would be taught . Now, perhaps because of the wider participation in higher education, the government wished to be assured that universities provided high quality teaching.

The National Committee of Inquiry into Higher Education (The Dearing Report) was published in April 1997. It had been commissioned by the UK government and was the largest review of higher education in the UK since the Robbins Committee in the early 1960s. The Dearing report put the student at the centre of the learning process with communication and information technologies in strong supporting roles. While this was supported by HEFCE, in the subsequent reorganisation Bristol lost its "Computers in Teaching Initiative Centre of Medicine" (CTICM) which had done so much to assist the Dental School establish its leading role in this field. However much of CTICM's expertise was absorbed into the new Institute for Learning and Teaching in Berkeley Square and with its help Bristol became the first school to deliver postgraduate teaching and CPD using teleconferencing.[168]

The Quality Assurance Agency for Higher Education (QAA) was established in 1997 and had been give the responsibility for assessing the quality of higher education (HE) in England and Northern Ireland from 1 October 1997 under the terms of a contract with the Higher Education Funding Council for England (HEFCE). In 1999 it carried out "Subject Reviews" aimed at ensuring that the public funding was supporting education of an acceptable quality, It did so under the headings of:

Curriculum Design, Content and Organisation.
Teaching, Learning and Assessment.
Student Progression and Achievement.
Student Support and Guidance.
Learning Resources.
Quality Management and Enhancement.

The visiting team of dental academics undertook direct observation of classroom, seminar and laboratory teaching, an assessment of the methods of reviewing students' work, and students' work itself. They examined the curriculum, methods of staff development, the application of resources (library, information technology, equipment), and student support and guidance. Each of these 6 areas was graded on a four-point scale (1 to 4), in ascending order of merit.

A huge amount of preparation was required for this exercise and the greater burden of the work was taken by Professor Harrison as Head of School and Dr. Robin Matthews the Clinical Dental Dean. Hundreds of man-hours were expended generating the required documentation. Suffice it to say that this filled an entire tutorial room which

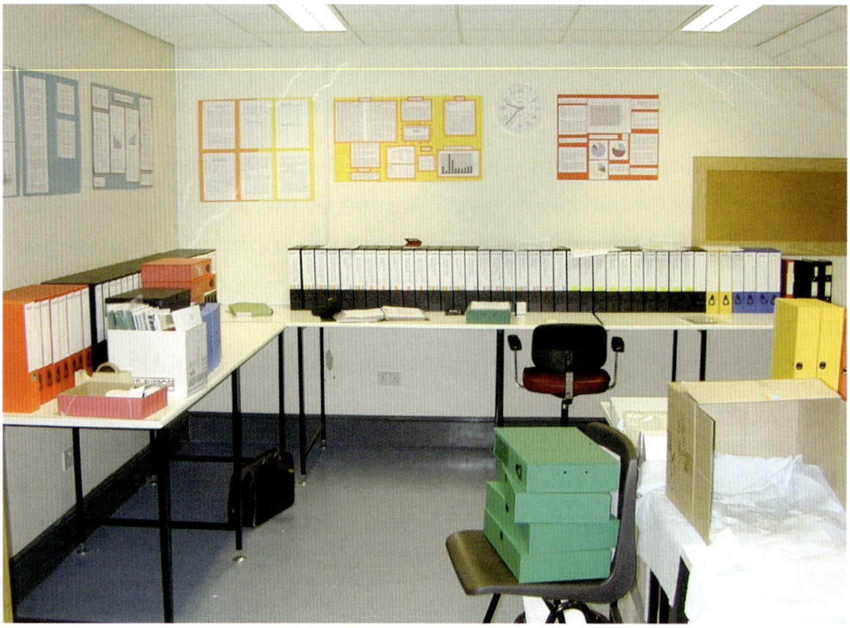

Figure 71. The School's teaching records in the "base room" ready for the HEFCE Teaching Review November 1999

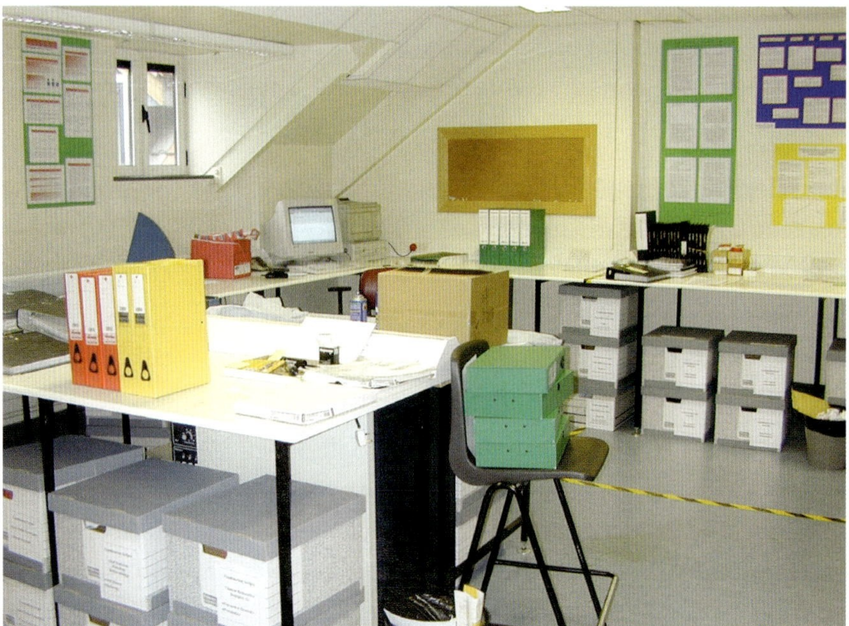

the visitors could have no more than glanced at.

The School was reviewed during the first two weeks in November 1999 and we were shocked to be judged as performing poorly in 4 out of the 6 assessments (our clinical medical colleagues fared little better!)[169] Nevertheless officially our 19/24 was regarded as "satisfactory" by the QAA, even so it was the lowest score in the University. There was a feeling of anger within the Dental School but a recognition that we had to be more formalized in our processes. We learnt that some schools had sufficient staff to be able to release a member of staff to spend six-months preparing their school's paperwork and had agreed and rehearsed their responses to likely questions.

Professor Jonathan Sandy, who had only recently been appointed as Chairman of the new Dental Education Committee, now took the lead in the dramatic improvement in the school's education monitoring processes .He said at the time:

> *"There is little doubt that the reviewers have provided us with clear direction as to how our teaching in dentistry needs to be improved. We believe that many of our weaknesses had previously been identified but that we lacked the infrastructure to make the changes necessary. We will improve and the collective spirit generated by the review process has done much to unite the school in an ambition to improve on all aspects even those which were not criticised".*

However in distinct contrast to this public response, privately school staff felt exactly as staff at other universities had done namely that such reviews should in future have a lighter touch and not involve the huge amount of paperwork, which the first review had necessitated.[170]

As with the case with the Research Assessment Exercise it was felt that with only 22 full time staff the School was ill equipped to provide the comprehensive input which the Teaching Review had demanded. In due course it was realized nationally that the review had been both expensive and unduly heavy handed.[171] Perhaps because of his prodigious efforts in the Teaching Review Robin Matthews decided it was time to move on and in March 1999 he accepted the chair in Oral Medicine in the University of the West Indies.

On Tuesday, September 28, 1999 , on the eve of her departure as President of the GDC, Margaret Seward had learnt to her great surprise that the Prime Minister would be announcing that day at the Labour party Conference in Bournemouth that by October 2001 anyone who wanted would be able to find an NHS dentist by telephoning NHS Direct.[172] [173] Shortly afterwards she became even more astonished to find herself appointed as Chief Dental Officer with the task of trying to achieve this admirable aim which would require an expansion of the UK dental undergraduate intake.

Chapter 10

ON INTO THE NEW MILLENNIUM

Uppermost in everyone's minds as we returned to the Dental School on 4th January 2000 was had our IT world been brought down by the "Millennium Bug" ? A huge amount of effort had been put into making sure all personal computers were Y2K compliant. Every machine in the school now had its little yellow sticker to show it have been checked. In the event everything performed normally.

In September 2000 the Government's Strategy to achieve the Prime Minister's election promises was announced.[174] There was considerable public doubt expressed about the dental strategy and just before Christmas the Parliamentary Health Committee announced an enquiry into whether this would improve dentistry in the long term.[175]

Alumni reunions were once again becoming a regular feature with a pattern of 5,10,15, 20 and 25 year reunions firmly established for almost all years. Most of these centred on old haunts but new ground had been broken in 1999 when one year met at Centre Parcs, Longleat. Later other years with young families adopted Alton Towers as their rendezvous. A highlight of many reunions has been the music provided by The Muskrats, a jazz band led by Reg Andlaw (Senior Lecturer Child Dental Health). He was a founder member of the band in 1992 and is now the sole surviver. An article about the band appeared in the Bristol Evening post in January 2004 and was reproduced in the 2004 issue of the newsletter of the Bristol Dental Alumni Association.

A number of people had retired or left in 1999, notably Sister/ Manager Yvie Theyer, Dr Neil Meredith and Louise Foster, the latter to take up the role of Dental Officer on the QE2 . Dr Mark Griffiths announced he would be leaving in May 2000 after 30 years at the school in a wide range of roles from conservation through oral medicine to special care dentistry.

Labour had come to power in 1997 with the slogan "Education, education, education!" This priority was to be reiterated in their re-election campaign of 2001, however it was made clear that the focus would remain primary and secondary education.[176]

The fallout from Subject Review was considerable. The reputation of the school was damaged although applications for places to study dentistry at Bristol were not diminished in any way. In fact applications to Bristol continued to increase despite the Subject Review score. Bristol is, after all, a wonderful place to study dentistry! Nevertheless 19/24 as a score (Medicine got 20/24) was the worst of all dental schools in the UK and was the worst Departmental score in the University of Bristol.

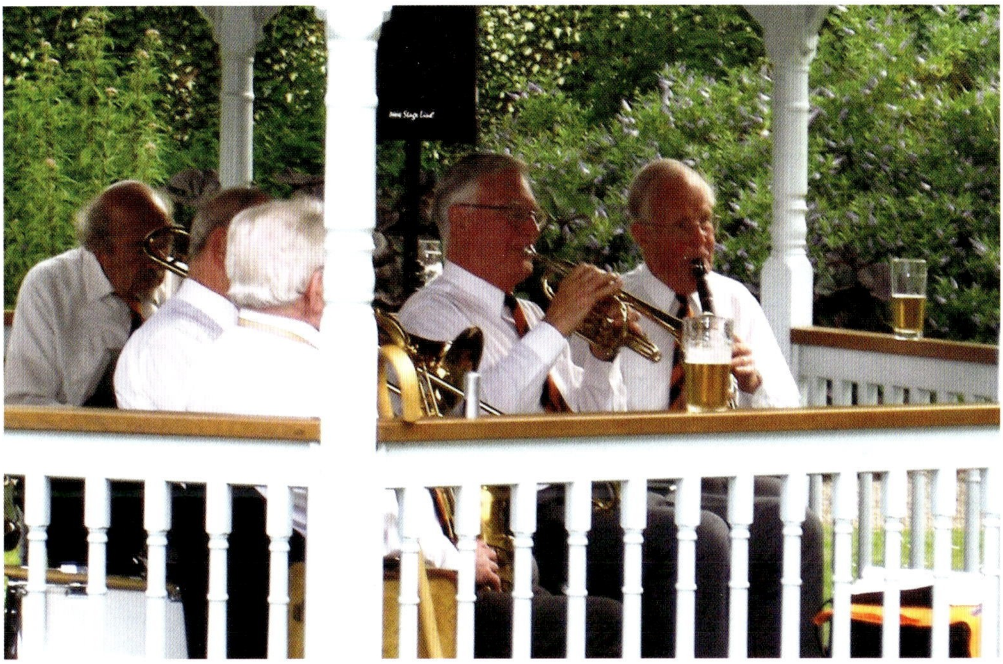

Figure 72. The Muskrats in 2009.

A great deal now needed to be done to ensure that our teaching process was judged outstanding when we were reassessed. Because of the universal criticism about the huge effort and cost of the original 1999 Quality Assurance Agency (QAA) review process this now became the responsibility of individual institutions. Jonathan Sandy who had received his personal chair in 1999 took on the crucial role of Chairman of the Dental Education Committee. All educational processes with the School were scrutinised in detail, areas of the curriculum were overhauled and codes of practice developed as a school-wide activity to ensure that our teaching could be shown to be "quality assured". The process now included the dental hygiene and surgery assistant courses in the Dental Care Professional (DCP)* School as well as all postgraduate programmes.

At the same time as the education processes were being overhauled, the School was having to prepare for the next Research Assessment Exercise for which the deadline for eligible output was December 2000. The stated aim of the Research Assessment Exercise (RAE) was to enable the higher education funding bodies to distribute public

* Several interesting accounts of these times are contained in Jerrard J. Reminiscences. University of Bristol Womens Club. Bristol,1997.

funds for research selectively on the basis of quality. Institutions conducting the best research would thus receive a larger proportion of the available funds. The results became known in December 2001. Bristol had 15 Departments scoring the highest grade of 5 compared with only 1 achieving this grade in 1996. Clinical dentistry was one of these 15 and the School's achievement was only equalled by Guys Hospital Dental School. In fact Bristol should be regarded as the best UK Dental School in this assessment since it had better International research returns than Guys. The achievement was not generally welcomed by our Bristol colleagues in Clinical Medicine who only scored 3a. A past dean of the Faculty went so far as to say that the clinical dentistry panel must have been applying different standards to that of clinical medicine! It is worth remembering that Bristol medicine had £18 million invested in it between the RAE of 1997 and 2001, while dentistry had received very little over the same period.

The initial rejoicing turned into a national furore when the HEFCE announced how the selectivity of research funding would be applied following a late decision by the Government to put no more money into university research. Only 5* scoring departments would now be level funded. Those scoring 5 would take a 15% cut and those scoring 3a would receive a 70% cut.[177, 178] The net result for Bristol's Faculty of Medicine was that while the Dental Cost Centre would receive an additional £137,000 p.a., the Vet School with a mere Grade 5 had a 15% cut and the Clinical Medical School (3a) had a 70% cut losing £1.2M. Bristol was not alone in this lunacy which came at a time when UK medical schools were being asked by government to increase their student intake!. As a result the Dental School, despite its huge efforts, gained not one penny in order to offset the deficit in the Bristol Medical Faculty as a whole.

The realisation by an impoverished University that more space would none the less have to be found for an increased medical student intake resulted in the decision by the United Bristol Hospitals Trust to build an Education Centre on the site adjacent to the Dental School on Upper Maudlin Street. Not for the first time did the Special Trustees, now known as the charity "Above and Beyond", come to the aid of the Trust and University. As with earlier developments we were able to watch the City's archaeologists at work on the site before building commenced.

The new Vice Chancellor Eric Thomas took office in September 2001. It was to our advantage that his daughter had recently completed a successful course of orthodontic treatment undertaken by a former Bristol postgraduate. He visited the Dental School personally, and was unaware of the unhappiness which the RAE outcome had caused. He promptly gave £100,000 to refurbish the dental clinical skills laboratory that in parts was 40 years old.

---

* DCP = dental nurse, hygienist, dental therapist, dental technician, orthodontic therapist and clinical dental technicians

In 2001 the Department of Clinical Medicine underwent an extensive review with external scrutiny from Sir Keith Peters and Sir John Savil. Professor Jonathan Sandy was asked to sit on the panel. After much discussion, the Vice Chancellor took the decision to split the existing Faculty into a Faculty of Medicine and Dentistry and a Faculty of Medical and Veterinary Sciences.

By this time Professor Stephen Lisney (BDS UBrist, 1975) the only dentist to become a Professor of Physiology had become Dean of the Faculty of Medicine (2000-2003). He it was who saw through the consequential changes in the faculty structure which now took place Such a changes were long overdue. The expectation that a clinical professor could run a Faculty which accounted for 40% of the University's expenditure on a part time basis in addition to his own departmental work was unreasonable. Indeed a few years before the professors in the Faculty had gone to the then Vice Chancellor Sir John Kingman asking forcibly that the Dean be made a full time free standing appointment; a request which was denied. The next incumbent was only in post for a few weeks before experiencing a heart attack.

There was now no doubt that two smaller Faculties would be more manageable and effective. A new full-time Dean of the Faculty of Medicine and Dentistry took office on 1st August 2003 and immediately undertook an academic review of all staff. This caused significant disruption and many staff felt very uneasy at having the quality of their research and their teaching activity evaluated. Clinical academics have always struggled more than most to fulfil the requirements of research, teaching and administration because of the additional burden of their clinical commitment. Given the financial climate it is difficult to know what else could have been done but this exercise caused a number of people to reflect on their positions at Bristol University.

In May 2002 Professor Raman Bedi (BDS UBrist 1976) was appointed CDO. It was a difficult time for UK dentistry which had just had its third Minister in 13 months. Two months later the long awaited "Options for Change" was published. The subsequent two years of negotiations can be read elsewhere[179] but in July 2004 John Reid, the Secretary of State for Health unveiled his plans for what would be the biggest reform in NHS dentistry since 1948. This was aimed at addressing the shortfall in NHS dental services. Dentistry as a whole would receive an additional £368m funding (a claimed increase of 19.3%).[180] Of more direct; importance to the Bristol Dental School was that there would to be a 25% increase in UK dental undergraduate places and places for dental therapists would be increased nationally from 50 to 200.

In 2003 the School underwent a routine General Dental Council inspection. Whilst there were still some areas which they felt needed attention there was much credit given for the rigorous quality assurance of education which was in place. In 2004 the

QAA undertook a new inspection of universities the so-called "Institutional Audit". The aim was to carry out a general inspection of the University processes and to examine selected departmental audit trials in detail. Clinical Medicine was supposed to have been the selected area for the Faculty of Medicine and Dentistry but the Vice Chancellor knew that Dentistry was now in much better shape (the Faculty had only just appointed a new Dean of Medicine and Dentistry) and so he telephoned HEFCE to request that dentistry be reviewed instead. Two dental programmes were examined: the BDS undergraduate programme and the orthodontic postgraduate programme (DDS). This was previously an MSc which had been adopted as a template for other orthodontic courses in the UK, but which at Bristol was now a professional doctorate. The reports on these two programmes were exemplary. A number of areas of good practice were identified which were subsequently described on the website of the Higher Education Academy's Learning and Teaching Support Network. Thus much had been done to rectify the poor performance in 1999 and to restore the reputation of the School.

When Raman Bedi received his Bristol LLD *honoris causa* in May 2003 informal discussions were already taking place as to how to achieve the proposed increase UK dental intake which John Reid had eventually announced in July 2004. Raman took the opportunity to ask if the School would be able accept another 20-30 students. He was told that as matters stood, the School did not have the staff, the space or a supply of patients to undertake this. He responded by saying that if this was not possible then the School would probably have to close, being seen as too small to be viable. The whole question of viability is an odd one and has been raised several times in recent years yet the basis on which viability is judged is never stated and was not on this occasion. It could not be on research output as we were only one of two HEFCE 5* rated UK dental schools. It could hardly be on teaching as two years before a survey of vocational trainees had ranked Bristol 4th from the top in adequacy of its undergraduate teaching[181] and we had just had an outstanding QAA review. .It could not be motivation of our students since at that time a higher percentage of Bristol dental graduates were achieving a postgraduate qualifications than in any other provincial dental school[182] (see Table opposite). All this had been achieved during a period when we had a higher student to staff ratio than any other UK dental school!

During the 1980s and 1990s the term "death by a thousand cuts" had become commonplace within universities. In the next decade the government's pursuit of "excellence" and "value for money" produced what can only be described as "distressment by assessment" for UK clinical academic staff. The situation was admirably described in 2004 by Friedy Luther (BDS UBrist,1984) a senior clinical lecturer at Leeds. She felt, as we all did, that eight school and personal assessments in two years was excessive.[183]

UNIVERSITY	Total graduates 1984 - 93	Those with PG qualifications	PG qualification %
Belfast	268	67	25.00
Birmingham	620	130	20.97
Bristol	386	112	29.02
Dundee	374	76	20.32
Edinburgh	398	95	23.87
England	824	226	27.43
Glasgow	551	103	18.69
Leeds	458	89	19.43
London	1968	579	29.42
Liverpool	490	101	20.61
Manchester	503	107	21.27
Newcastle	642	145	22.59
Sheffield	408	61	14.95
Wales	356	85	23.88
National total	8246	1976	23.96

Figure 73. An analysis by university of registered additional postgraduate dental qualifications achieved by UK dental graduates for the ten-year registration period 1984 to 1993 (N =8246).

While the pressures on dental academic posts had by now been widely recognised[184, 185, 186] nothing was put in place to improve matters. Bristol's list of assessments was almost identical to that of Leeds but in addition, the GDC's visit in 2003 had produced the recommendation that we should review our BDS curriculum. This review was begun in 2004, but this was soon followed by the request to "consider" increasing our undergraduate numbers which rendered obsolete the work on the curriculum up to that date.

A notable undergraduate success during this difficult period was that Gordon Carey became the UK Dentsply student clinician of 2002. (Sadly his travel to Kansas to take part in the international competition was cancelled due to the 9/11 Twin Towers disaster). This was followed by Angela Nobbs, a PhD student in Oral Microbiology, who won the Unilever research poster prize at the British Society for Dental Research meeting in Belfast. The following year Jeremy Peak (BDS UBrist,1989) became the UK young businessman of the year in a competition sponsored by HSBC, Sky News and the Daily Express. After the GDC elections of 2003 three Bristol graduates found themselves on the Council: David Philips (BDS,1965); John Chope (BDS,1972) and David Keetly (BDS,1985); more than any other school could claim.

As is always the case in dynamic schools, able and ambitious staff are head hunted and gain promotion elsewhere. In time of University cutbacks, such vacancies are immediately frozen pending a case being made for their replacement. In 2002 Dr. Klaus Jandt departed for a chair in Biomaterials in his native Germany and Alison Williams moved to a new chair in Health Services Research at GKT.[187] Richard Vowles the unsung hero of the Computer Assisted Learning Room took over many of the dental material lectures in the following months. To these staff losses were soon added the retirements of Professor Alan Harrison and Dr David Williams from Prosthetics, Derek Coles from Oral Medicine and Dental Instructor Richard Garn. These last three had spent almost all of their professional lives at the School. Finally Jeremy Rees who had done so much to see the new technique lab with its phantom head simulator officially opened by the Vice Chancellor in March 2004 departed a month later for a Chair in Restorative Dentistry at Cardiff.

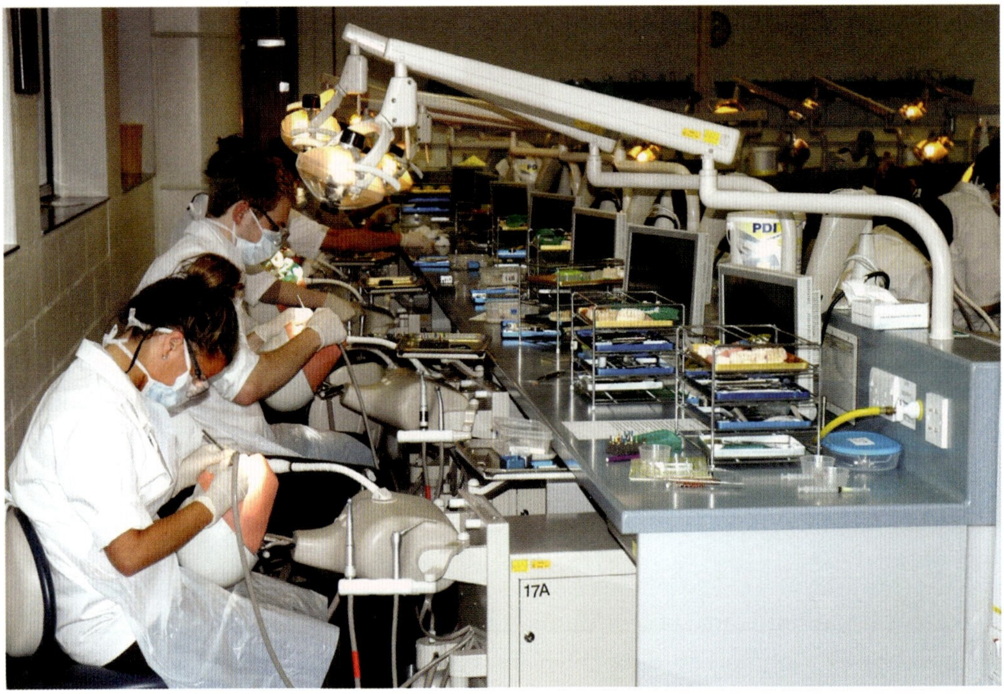

Figure 74. The refurbished Phantom head room (2010) in the 1985 extension.

As well as these staff losses, structural alterations were soon to take place in the building. At this challenging time Professor Steve Prime took over as Head of School. It is a huge credit to the determination and cohesion of the staff that students remained almost completely unaware of these pressures although not the structural changes. As the student president observed in 2007 "at times a hard hat seemed more appropriate than a white coat".[188] Yet by 2009 Bristol was identified by students as the best place in the UK to study dentistry. This information was derived from the national student survey [NSS] which had become one of the measures by which the government had decided all universities and departments should be judged.[189] It had taken a decade to overcome the poor position in 1999 when we were viewed as the worst department in the University of Bristol.

In 2010 we remained the best dental school in England. In the same two years the School was to be found among best 5% of departments in the University of Bristol. As a further indication of the quality of dental teaching Faculty Teaching Awards were made in that year to David Dymock, Dominic O'Sullivan, Susan Hooper, Gordon Gray, Michele Barbour, Angela Hague and Jonathan Sandy. Susan Hooper was voted DDU teacher of the year in 2009, preceded by Alison Grant from the DCP School in 2008. In 2010 Stephen Lisney and Nikki Rogers now cleaned up with the DDU awards for best Dental and best DCP teachers respectively. The following year Susan Hooper had been awarded a prestigious University Teaching Fellowship and finally David Dymock was appointed Faculty Education Director for a 3 year term where no doubt his experience of teaching in Dentistry will benefit medical teaching.

The agreement in 2004 to greatly expand the dental intake at Bristol had been based on the belief that money would be provided for increased clinical facilities and in October 2005 the Bristol dental undergraduate intake rose from 55 to 86. It was reduced slightly the following year to 75 plus 4 overseas students (total intake 79), when the Department of Health decided to establish the Peninsula Dental School. Even so the final increase at Bristol was still the largest of any UK dental school but as yet the clinical facilities remained those for a school of 55 clinical students! News of the success of the joint bid from the University and the United Bristol Healthcare Trust (UBHT) for funding for the additional clinical facilities came in June 2007 to great

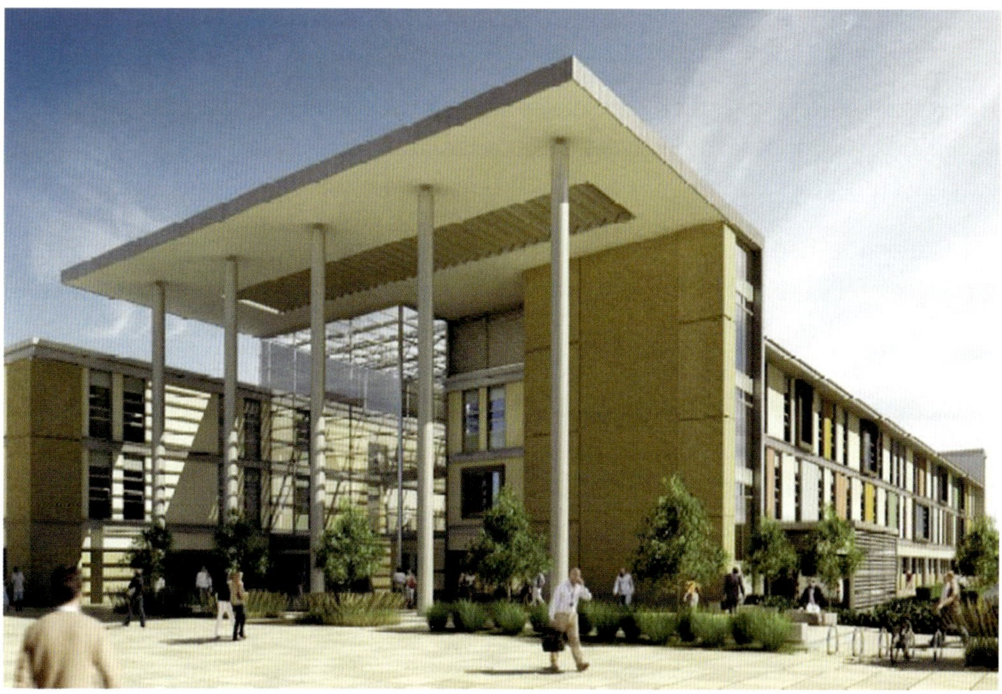

Figure 75. An artist's impression of the South Bristol Community Hospital.

relief all round. This secured £13,137,000 in capital investment from the Department of Health, and £2,200,000 capital from the Higher Education Funding Council for England. The increased revenue would come from the increased student numbers but it was soon realised that the capital was essentially a mortgage, which would have to be paid back through continued income generation. Some staff were sceptical as to whether promised increased staffing would come about and whether student numbers might at some point be reduced again. If this were the case how would the school generate the income that was needed to pay off these loans?

The expansion was heavily dependent on a dental outreach clinic being built in south Bristol. The School had some experience of operating an outreach clinic at the Charlotte Keel Health Centre. As in other UK dental schools this practice was highly valued by students. It had been agreed that a 12 chair dental unit would be provided in the "soon to be constructed" South Bristol Hospital. Inevitably there has been delay and when the increased clinical intake arrived at the School work on this not started but it is hoped that this new facility will come on stream in September 2012.

As Rushton and Horner succinctly observed:

> *"Paradoxically, to the external eye, an observer might interpret the recent expansion in UK undergraduate numbers as evidence of a thriving and expanding academia. In fact, this expansion is taking place in the absence of a concomitant expansion in the number of academic staff. Furthermore, the new English dental schools are following a path of clinical teaching in the community and relying on a very small core of trained academics."* [190]

This was absolutely true and by now in Bristol, as in all other dental schools, about 50% of clinical teaching was undertaken by honorary university staff (visiting consultants, specialist registrars, community dental officers and general dental practitioners).

The DCP school had also undergone significant changes. For many years this had been run successfully under the leadership of Sheila Lockyer. When she retired there was an opportunity to consider closer integration between the DCP training and the dental undergraduate curriculum. It was also thought appropriate to develop programmes for therapists, hygienists and clinical dental technicians in line with the thinking of the Department of Health. Sarah Bain now took over the leadership of the DCP school and when Martin Woodhead (Consultant in Restorative Dentistry) retired, Jonathan Sandy took over as Director of the DCP school from 2005 to 2008 whereupon Sarah Bain then became the first DCP to be appointed as a Director of a UK DCP School.

The DCP school now became fully integrated in the new undergraduate curriculum which focussed on to developing team working. Three new DCP programmes were begun: a hygiene/therapy program, a therapy program for hygienists wishing to convert to dental therapy and an orthodontic therapy programme, because as mentioned earlier Bristol had piloted an such a programme in the 1990s.[191] The DCP School in Bristol is now the largest provider of DCP training in the United Kingdom. All programmes were visited by the GDC from 2008 onwards and all were deemed "sufficient".

Professor Stephen Prime completed his three-year term as Head of School in 2007 and was succeeded by Professor Jonathan Sandy who was appointed for a four year term).

The research profile of the school was also changing. A long-term view had been taken and the decision made to invest in research staff in the field of oral health. This meant not replacing Chris Stephens and Alison Williams from orthodontics and a lecturer post from oral and maxillofacial surgery. Professor Ness (Epidemiology) was appointed to lead this new research group assisted by a nutritionist (Charlotte Atkinson) a statistician (Sam Leary), a psychologist (Andrea Waylen) and a health economist (Melissa Ke). Although this group was not returned in the 2008 RAE for dentistry, in the 2008 RAE Bristol was positioned 5th of all dental schools in the UK with a much greater proportion of "research active staff" returned than in 2001.

During 2008 the School also underwent a Departmental Review, now a regular part of the University review process. The refurbishment of the Dental Hospital had been completed by this time and the facilities were judged to be excellent. A significant number of recommendations were made by the University and this was also an opportunity for the Department to voice its concerns about the recent increase in student numbers which had been made without any commensurate increase in staffing.[192]

Following the review a restructuring of the Hospital and School was undertaken. As a result all Teaching Divisions were removed and the Department now operates as a single unit. This was far sighted as two years later the University as a whole underwent restructuring with the elimination of departments and we were able to move from a Department of Oral and Dental Sciences to a School of Oral and Dental Sciences with very little further change in structure. By now the University was starting to experience significant financial pressures brought about by 2008 economic slowdown. Inevitably research activity came under significant scrutiny and it was decided that unfunded research and 2* (national significance only) research could not continue. The research at the School was reorganized into three groupings, oral health, microbiology and biomaterials. The research income which in the period 2001-2008 had been approximately £6 million has now increased significantly to more than £13 million during 2008 to 2011. Current grant income includes seven awards for more than £250,000 and four awards of over £1 million.

The staffing increases at this time (in addition to those described above associated with the appointment of Professor Ness) have included Nicky Kilpatrick (Professor in Paediatric Dentistry), Steve Thomas (Professor in Oral and Maxillofacial Surgery) Nicola

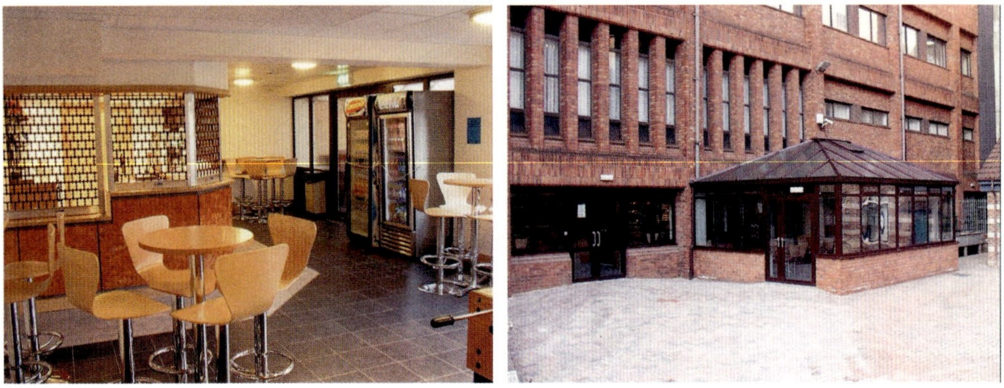

Figure 76. The reprovision of the Students Common Room and bar in 2008 which the Alumni supported financially.

West (Professor in Restorative Dentistry) Dominic O'Sullivan (Professor in Restorative Dentistry) Crispian Scully (Professor in Oral Medicine), Nigel Robb (Reader in Restorative Dentistry) Jim Middleton (Reader in Immunology) Miranda Pring (Senior Lecturer in Oral and Maxillo-Facial Pathology), Nicola Cirillo (Lecturer in Oral Medicine), Carla Fleming (Lecturer in Oral Surgery), Barry Maine (Lecturer in Oral and Maxillofacial Surgery), Rhena Bhat (Paediatric Teaching Fellow), Angela Nobbs (Lecturer in Microbiology). In addition consultant posts have been achieved in Radiology (Jane Luker and Rebecca Davies), Special Needs Dentistry (Tony Brooke) Oral and Maxillofacial Surgery (Ceri Hughes) and Paediatric Dentistry (Sarah Dewhurst). These have been part funded by the University in recognition of teaching needs. Bo Su and Tony Ireland received internal promotion to Readerships, Sam Leary, Charlotte Atkinson and Michele Barbour internal promotion to Senior Lecturerships. Appointments at all levels were difficult because of the National shortage of academics prepared to work in Dental schools. Retirements included Christ Stephens, Alan Harrison, Ken Marshall and John Eveson. Jon Cowpe and Daryll Jagger moved to further their careers elsewhere.

The establishment in 2006 of the National Institute of Health Research by the Department of Health has provided for the first time a means of addressing and funding UK health service research priorities. This move aimed at establishing a health research system in which the NHS supports outstanding individuals in world-class facilities who can conduct leading-edge research focussed on the needs of patients and the public. This support also included NIHR Clinical Lectureships, specialty training posts that incorporate academic training, to address what has now been recognised by government as an acute shortage of academic trainees. As a School, Bristol did really well following the introduction of this new scheme. The first academic clinical fellow appointed was Helen Petersen (BDS, U.Brist, 2005) and within nine months she was awarded a Wellcome Trust Research Training Fellowship. A further Bristol graduate Holly Cole-Hawkins (BDS, U.Brist, 2008) has been awarded an NIHR Research Training Fellowship and a further academic clinical fellow has been granted an interview for a Wellcome Trust Research Training Fellowship. The award of an NIHR Biomedical Research Unit to Professor Andy Ness (£5.5 million) is unprecedented in dentistry in the UK. These achievements in research have not been seen in the Dental School for the last twenty years.

The first decade of the 21st century saw the retirements or movements from the School of many loyal staff: Ann Jones, Sally Gregg, Pauline Ford Jennie Beddoe and Sarah Smith. In 2011 the University decided to restructure finance, personnel and academic support. This meant the further loss of staff who had provided long service to the School and University. The consequential loss of corporate memory may have a significant effect as the school moves forward and other avenues of support will have to be found.

Chapter 11

STUDENT RETROSPECT AND PROSPECT

Without dental students there would be no dental school. In recent years Bristol has been able to attract students of the highest calibre and of a wide social mix. The Student Society has been responsibly and ably led by a series of outstanding Presidents. It was an inspired move when in the mid 1970s the student body decided that their president should be elected from the penultimate year of the course rather

1942	J.V. Gibson	1977	D.G.Lammond
1943	J.F.Woolley	1978	M.J.Fardy
1944		1979	G.E.Mendham
1945	P.J.Blyth	1980	G.Shovlin
1946		1981	K.Hemmings
1947	A.J.P Cousins	1982	D.E.Wood
1948	R.T.Jones	1983	J.P.Baber
1949	C.H.Thomas	1984	K.R.Ferguson
1950	D.McAndlish	1985	I.A.Allan
1951	M.R.Treweeke	1986	R.J.Spencer
1952	A.J.Drinnan	1987	T.J.Sunnocks
1953		1988	C.B.Whitewhead
1954	D.Kalra	1989	C.J Dunham
1955	D.J.Harries	1990	Kellie Solino
1956	MJ Garry	1991	Sarah Sobrian
1957	A.J.Moore	1992	Tamara Khayatt
1958	D.R.James	1993	Stephenie Wilkin
1959	G.Duggan	1994	Colin Langley
1960	D.M.Treharne	1995	Alison Brokenshire
1961	J.E.Sheid	1996	Andrew Bain
1962	P. Sayzeland	1997	James Gabriel
1963	F.A.Leach	1998	Gary Price
1964	D.C.Lewis	1999	Paul McGannity
1965	J.Lucia	2000	Gary Porter
1966	I.L.Kelly	2001	Rishi Patel
1967	P.J.Richardson	2002	James Granger
1968	R.C.Miller	2003	Goldie Songra
1969	J.N.Spaven	2004	Ediz Cakin
1970	I.A.Grant	2005	Michael Lessani
1971	R.T.Mallenson	2006	Jennifer Moorcroft
1972	C.V.Lansley	2007	Adam Radford
1973	D.M.Adlam	2008	Christoph Harper
1974	S.B.Kneebone	2009	Sarah Buckley
1975	Catherine Asher	2010	Hajirah Mir
1976	S.A.Gooda		

Figure 77. The UBDSS Presidents.

than the final year. No longer was a student president highly likely to fail his or her finals but instead was able in the final year to advise a successor. For their leadership it seems only right to record here the student presidents who have contributed so much in the past and have often gone on to provide a valuable point of contact for year reunions. In doing so it is recognised that the Secretary of the Student Society in each year usually made an equal contribution.

Reunions have been a feature of the School's graduates, surely in indication of enjoyable time spent at Bristol. These have been nurtured and encouraged both before and since his retirement by Dr. Reg Andlaw. Of the last 46 years of graduates all but 6 now have regular reunions.

Individual years have their own unique character and talents but there are common threads running through the generations. The first has to be football both traditional and table football. In the latter the record must go to Barry Gilling and Phil Ratcliffe who were medal winners in all four years in the Annual Bristol Dental Hospital Table Football Competitions between 1971 and 1975.

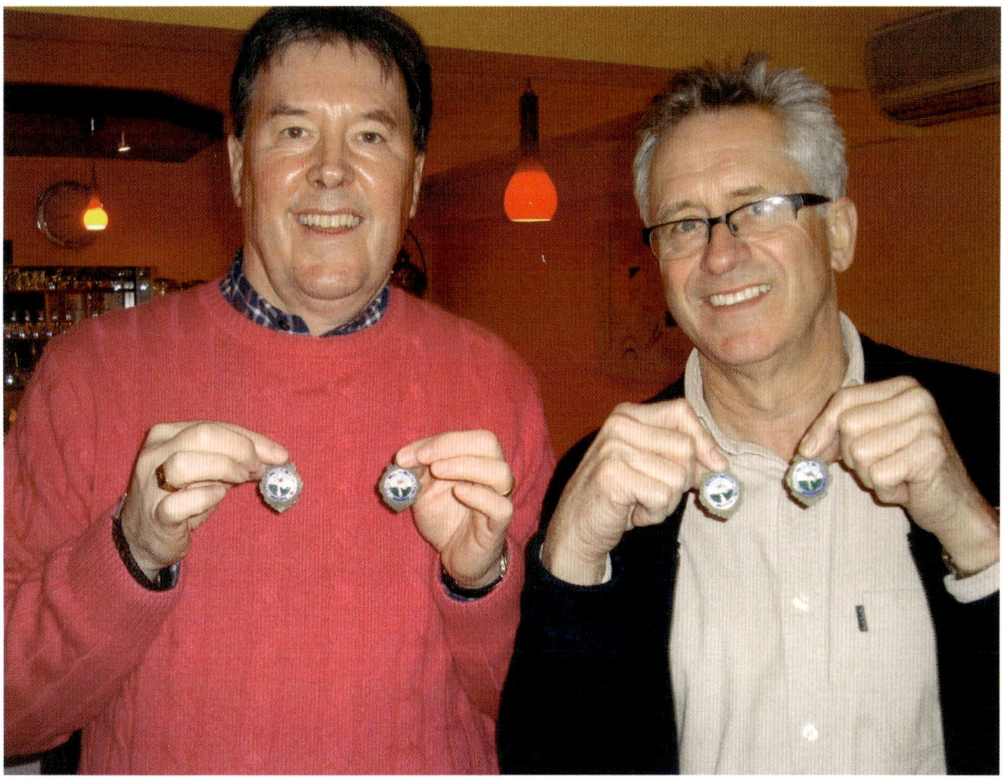

Figure 78. Barry Gilling and Phil Ratcliffe "We practised for hours" (*but not at dentistry*).

There are many other examples of the extramural skills of students coming to enrich life in the Dental School.

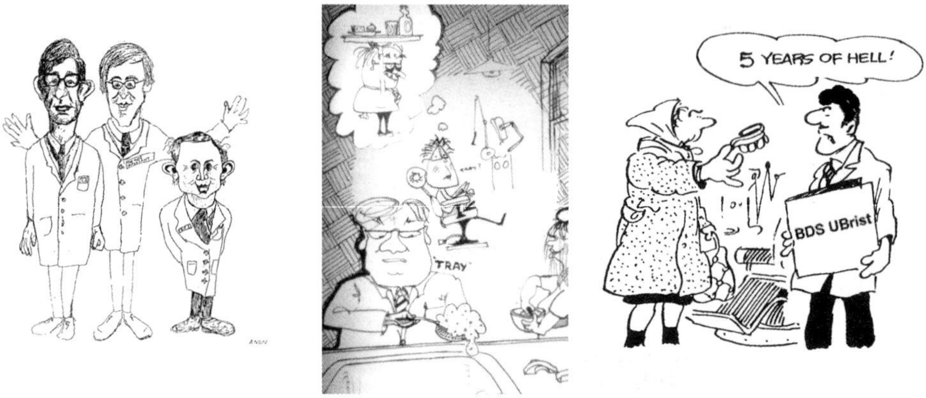

Figure 79. Various student cartoons.

There have been athletes and actors, runners and writers, cartoonists and cricketers, sportswomen and singers, musicians and mountaineers and these are only the few which we know about. Only one year produced a chamber orchestra, and as far as we know only one student, Geoff Downer (BDS UBris, 1976), produced a book as an undergraduate. His popular "Illustrated Guide to Dental Morphology" is sadly now out of print but a second hand copy currently commands a £40 price!

There are many student traditions at Bristol that have stood the test of time.

The Hannover Exchange

As far as is known, this is unique amongst UK dental schools and around 480 dental students from Bristol have benefited from the experience it has provided over the past 38 years.

The impetus came from Professor Bradford in 1971 , who felt that the Dental School should follow the lead set by the Veterinary School whose link with the Veterinary University in Hannover, Bristol's twinned city in Germany. This had been successfully in existence since the late 1940's. The task of investigating and establishing a similar dental contact was delegated to Ken Marshall, one of Professor Bradford's lecturing staff. The first problem was that there was no evidence of a dental school in Hannover so it was decided that Ken, with one of the senior dental students, should join that year's veterinary exchange group so that the situation could be explored. It transpired that the Dental School in Hannover was about to move from temporary accommodation into brand new building within the Hannover Medical University complex. Professor Jung of the Hannover School was keen to participate in the proposed link and it was agreed that exchange visits would be delayed until the new Dental School in Hannover was occupied. The first party of senior students, from Bristol under the leadership of Professor Bradford made the trip to Hannover in 1973. The pattern of

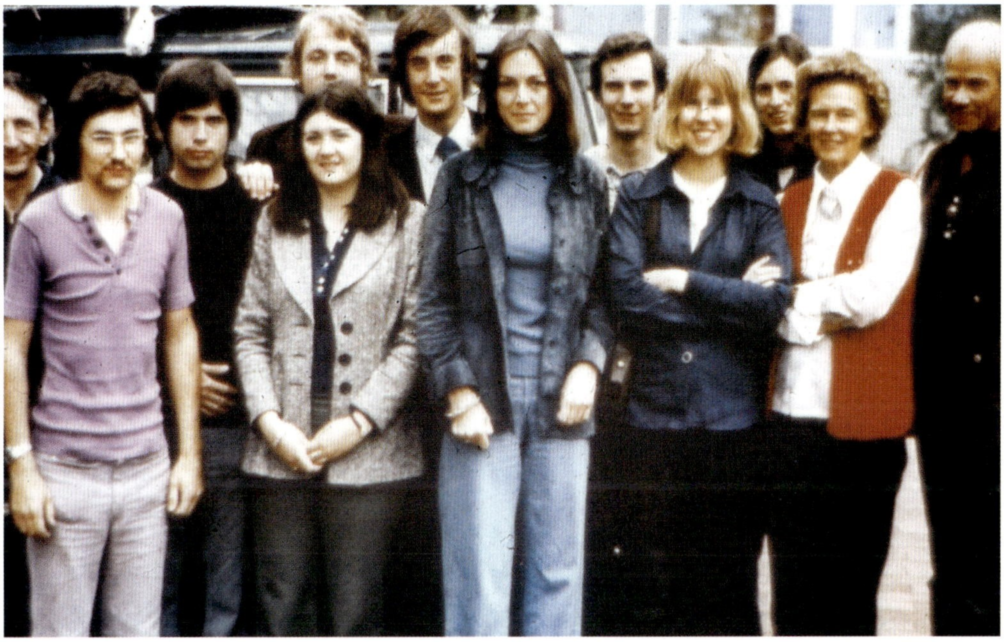

Figure 80. The 1973 Hanover exchange. Jacqueline Masterson, fourth from the right, later became a house officer at Hannover.

the exchange visit followed the veterinary example, enabling the Bristol contingent not only to compare all aspects of the two Dental Schools but also to experience the lifestyle differences that Germany had to offer. It also followed the veterinary example in agreeing that future annual exchanges would be one way only, with each of the Schools alternating in strict rotation as hosts.

Probably the most surprising discovery was the great similarity between the curricula and practices of the two schools However in the 1970's German dental students tended to be much older than their counterparts in the UK. Dentistry was considered to be the most desirable profession to enter in Germany, even exceeding medicine in this respect, and prospective students were prepared to remain on a waiting list for several years in order to gain entry. This has changed over the years, probably due to the increasing number of dental places in Germany.

The first thirty years of the exchange have concentrated on establishing firm staff links and raising the funds to support the cultural aspects. The latter task was made all the easier by the efforts of interested staff in both Schools and the fact that many dental manufacturing and supply companies were enjoying a period of expansion in their business and were in a position to lend generous support through sponsorship of the exchange programme events.

Although the senior students have, over the years, been the principal beneficiaries of the exchange scheme there have also been significant staff exchanges and interaction. During the waiting period for the Hannover School to be completed and prior to the first student exchange, it was agreed that an exchange of staff would take place and this involved a member of the lecturing staff in conservative dentistry from each of the Schools. Also, one of the1976 Bristol graduates spent time in Hannover as a House Officer in Restorative Dentistry. Since then the main obstacle to the continuation of exchanges, as might be expected, has been language proficiency. Around the turn of the Millennium, however, staff links became more active again when Professor Rossbach the then Dean of Hannover Dental School was appointed as an external examiner for the Final BDS in Bristol and one of his lecturers came to Bristol to study for a PhD.

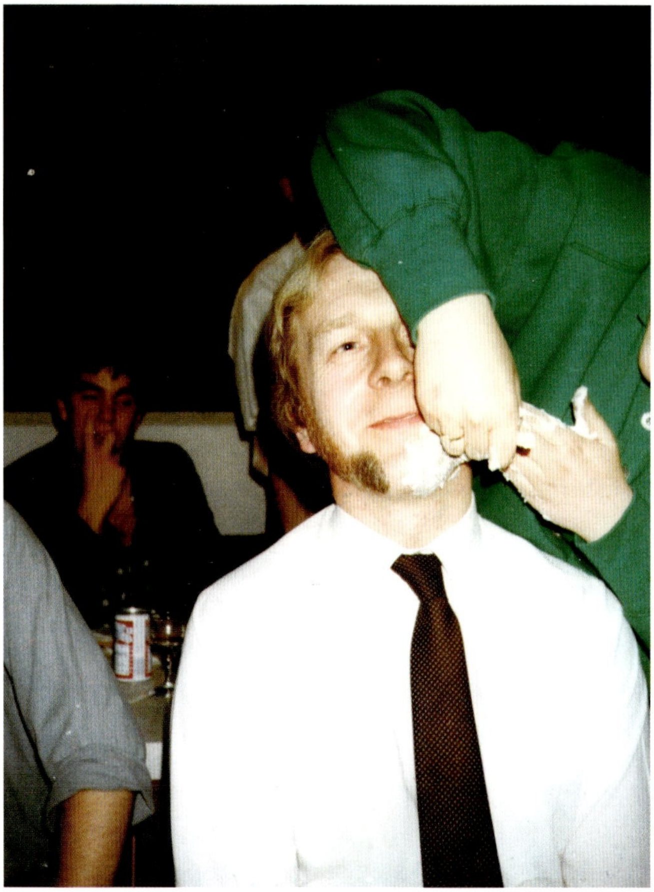

Figure 81. Martin Woodhead loses his sideburns in 1987 in aid of the Hannover Exchange.

The Student Show

The availability of the Nurses Teaching Unit in 1975 transformed the "Smoker" from a rude random happening into a full scale pantomime, written and directed by Ken Marshall. This was the first of a series of well written and rehearsed shows which were both clean and amusing. Some of the later ones were videoed by Ken Cowles and sold in aid of student funds. One wonders if any copies are still in existence.

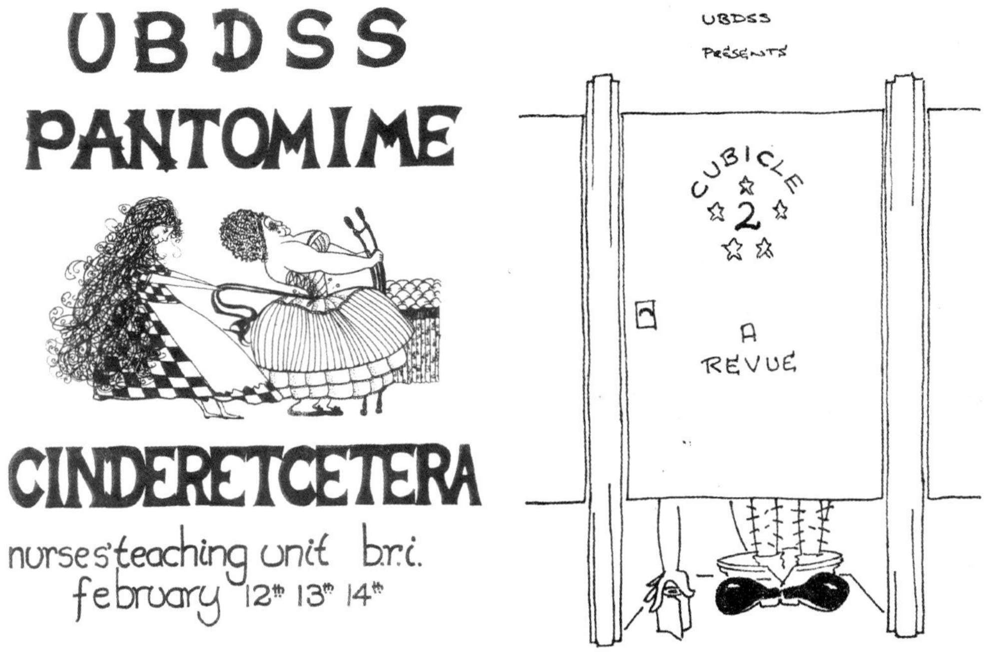

Figure 82. The 1975 and 1979 Student Show programmes.

The Final Year Dinner

The final year dinner has been in existence, probably from the time when Arthur Darling arrived in Bristol as it follows the pattern which exists at Newcastle. All students and staff attend this on the evening prior to the announcement of the final BDS results. The pre dinner drinks are usually sponsored by the Bristol Dental Alumni Association. Dental Defence Organisations make other contributions in the hope of signing up members the following day while the Final Year is still recovering from their generosity.

The Dental Ball

Until 1974 there was no formal occasion where staff, nurses and students in all years could attend. That all changed with the arrival of the Dental Ball at the Holiday Inn (now the Marriott Hotel City Centre), then the largest hotel in Bristol. Then Student

Committee took a huge risk. Such an event had not been attempted before and there were a great deal of up front costs. How many people would attend? What would happen if they did not? In the event it was a remarkable success and with an attendance of 300. It even made a profit ensuring that the Dental Ball is still regular annual event in the student year.

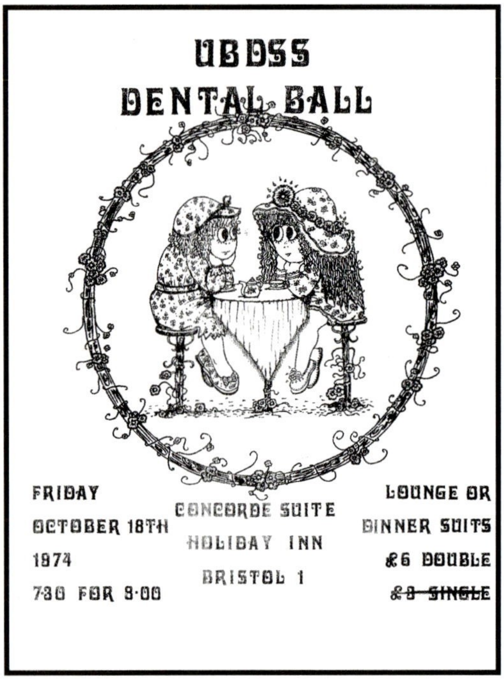

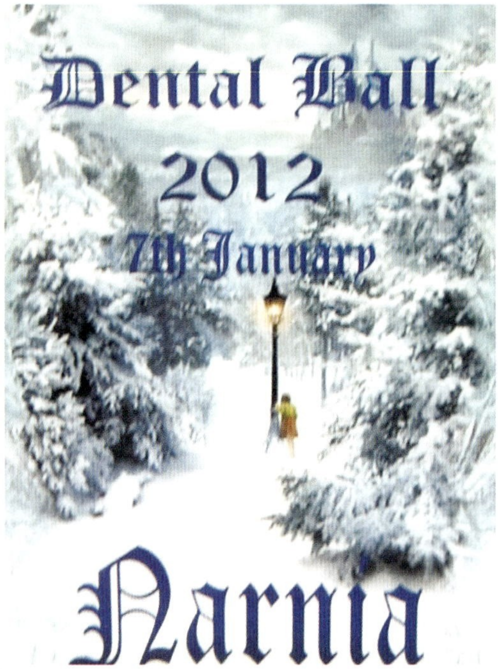

Figure 83. (a) The first UBDSS Ball in 1974; (b) still going strong in 2012.

The recent increase in the size of the School and the sharp increase in student fees to £9,000 pounds per annum are bound to impact on the character of the School. Increasing reliance on computer based teaching and less tutorial time are likely to weaken the social structure of the School. On the other hand, as pointed out in Chapter 10, the Bristol Dental School has an outstanding teachers as shown by its unequalled record in the DDU "Dentist teacher of the Year" awards. Nevertheless there is no place for complacency and in an increasingly competitive world a strong Dental Student Committee and Dental Alumni Association will be essential in maintaining the social life of the School which so many of us have enjoyed and in meeting future corporate and financial challenges. The author urges that anyone reading this who is not already a member of the Bristol Dental Alumni Association should join at once. Subscription forms are available from the Clinical Dean's Office and also downloadable from the Alumni website. Donations to Alumni funds are of course welcome at any time!

APPENDIX 1

PROFESSOR ARTHUR DARLING CBE - A PERSONAL PERSPECTIVE

Professor Chris Stephens

Arthur was a proud Northumberland man, one of his ancestors had been Grace Darling, and he showed the same energy and grit. While an undergraduate he had come under the influence of Robert Bradlaw, later Sir Robert Bradlaw, who became President of the General Dental Council and was the leading figure in mid 20th century UK dentistry. Quite apart from his professional achievements and influence Bradlaw was much loved by his staff and students both at Newcastle and later at the Eastman Dental Institute. Four "Bradlaw boys" from his time at Newcastle were in due course to become deans of UK dental schools and all of them endeavoured to emulate their mentor. Arthur was no exception yet his innate brusqueness was to be a handicap. His namesake Robert Alexander Darling, who was no relation, found himself applying for a place to study dentistry at Newcastle where Arthur was already a student. At his interview Robert was told that one disruptive Darling was enough for any dental school and he was dismissed without be able to say a word.[193]

Unlike many young would be academics I had never met Arthur Darling until my interview at Bristol in 1971. Had I done so I would not have applied for the post. At the time, unbeknown to me, he was renowned as a fearsome and belligerent examiner in the Dental Fellowship of the Royal College of Surgeons of England to the extent that many based in the south of England chose to take the Edinburgh Fellowship to avoid humiliation. The story is told of how a post-war ex services candidate having been goaded by Arthur in a viva voice examination rose to his feet and towering above his tormentor said "I have killed better men than you!" and strode out of the exam. Although all this was unknown to me at the time senior colleagues did advise me darkly to think very carefully before accepting an appointment at Bristol. To me though the attraction of Bristol at the time was its first class undergraduate course. It was said to me by a colleague who had taught in several UK schools that you could organise a dental school in three ways: for the benefit of patients, the staff or the students. Bristol was certainly in the last group.

There is no doubt that in his early years at Bristol Arthur was a titan – intelligent, determined and immensely energetic. However when he was appointed in 1947 at the age of 29 as the first Professor of Dental Surgery and Director of Dental Education at Bristol, his blunt northern approach did not go down well with senior hospital and faculty colleagues.

It was perhaps inevitable that soon after his arrival he would fall out with his hospital

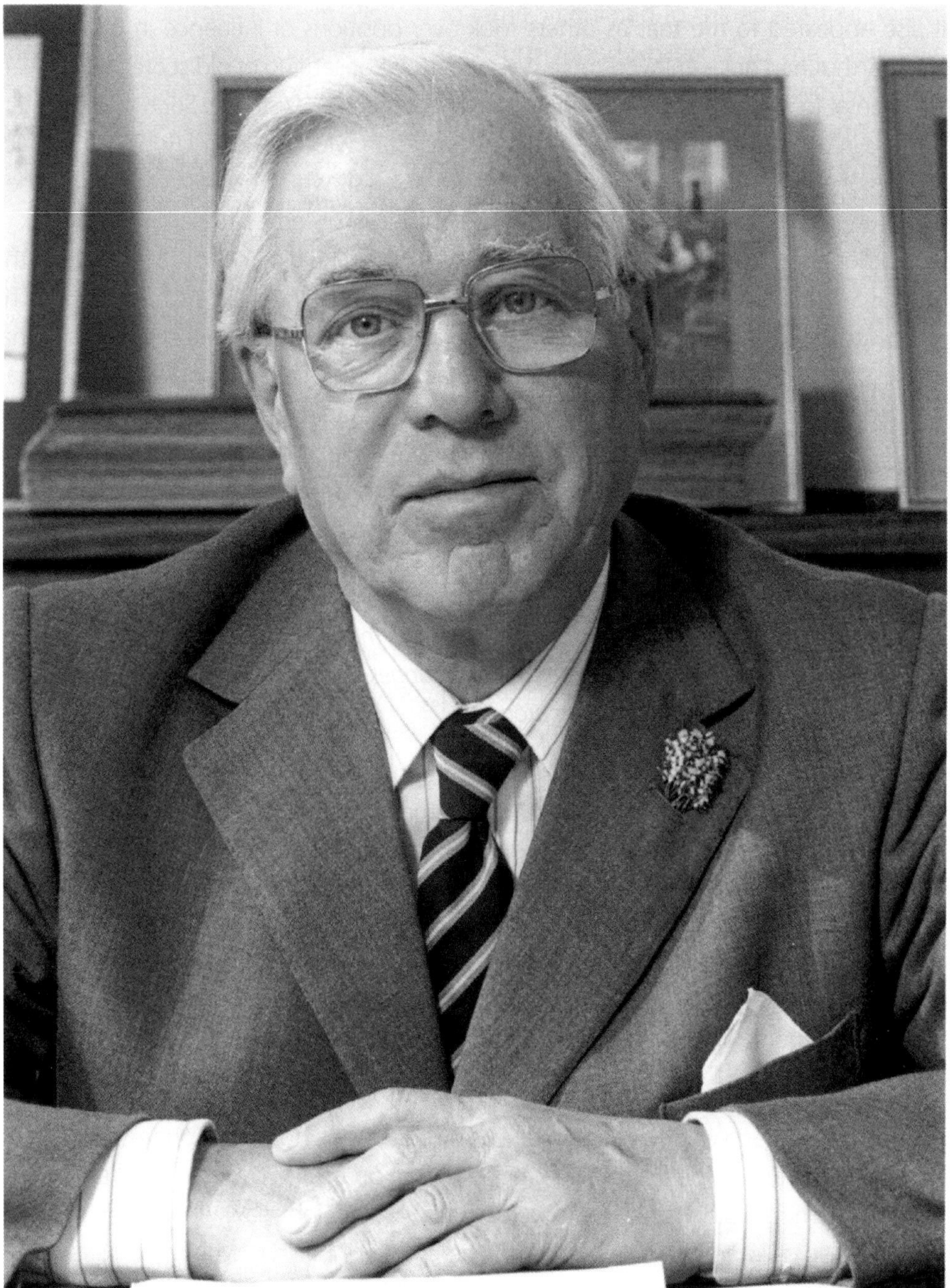

Figure 84. Professor Arthur Darling CBE, MRCS, LRCP, MDS, DDSc, FDSRCSEng in July 1982.

APPENDIX 2

DENTAL STAFF AT BRISTOL 1894-1988

Dental Lecturers Of The Medical School (1876-1893) and University College (1894-1910)

The dental staff of the University College, the General Hospital and the Infirmary were appointed independently. However in such a small field many held appointments in more than one institution during their professional lives. Thus Cooke Parsons, dental surgeon at the Bristol General Hospital was the first Lecturer in Dental Surgery at University College. He later became its Lecturer in Dental Mechanics in 1889 by relinquishing his earlier appointment in favour of William Ackland who was dental surgeon at the Bristol Infirmary.

THOMAS COOKE PARSONS	1876-1892	Lecturer Dental Mechanics later Dental Surgery
MR COOMBER	1877-1893	Lecturer in Dental Metallurgy
MR COE AND MR TIBBITS	1877-1889	Lecturers in Dental Surgery
CHARLES A HAYMAN	1893-1914	Lecturer in Dental Mechanics. Dental Metallurgy until 1909
WILLIAM R ACKLAND	1889-1922	Lecturer in Dental Mechanics later Dental Surgery
LOUIS EDMUND CLAREMONT	1922-1929	Lecturer in Dental Surgery
AUGUSTUS W W HOFFMAN	1894-1895	Lecturer in Dental Metallurgy
PROF A F STANLEY KENT	1899-1918	Lecturer in Physiology & Dental Anatomy.
0 C M DAVIS	1902-1942	Lecturer in Dental Materia Medica
EDWARD A DOWLING	1907-1922	Dental Anatomy, Physiology & Dental Histology

BRISTOL GENERAL HOSPITAL DENTAL STAFF 1874-1940

Dental Surgeons

THOMAS COOKE PARSONS	1874-1890
THOMAS TAYLOR GEORGE	1890-1907
EDWARD ALFRED DOWLING	1908-1922
LOUIS EDMUND CLAREMONT	1922-1929
NORMAN HAROLD KETTLEWELL	1929-1940
SYDNEY KILSHAW RIGG	1930-1940

Assistant Dental Surgeons

H J WYATT	1911-1923
S K RIGG	1923-1930
N H KETTLEWELL	1923-1929
E K TRATMAN	1926-1930
I G SUTHERLAND	1930-1932
F R HOGBIN	1930-1940
J WELLS	1932-1940

BRISTOL INFIRMARY DENTAL STAFF 1888-1940

Dental Surgeons

WILLIAM ROBERT ACKLAND	1888-1922
FREDERICK CECIL NICHOLS	1922-1940

Assistant Dental Surgeons

CHARLES AUGUSTUS HAYMAN	1904-1909
FREDERICK CECIL NICHOLS	1909-1922
GEORGE FREDERICK FAWN	1922-1940

1940-1950

Lecturers, Tutor and Recognised Teachers

N H KETTLEWELL	G F FAWN
W J LENNOX	P J STOY
R B PICKLES	R H MCKEAG

Senior Registrar

D GIBSON DAVIES

Registrar

R S SAXTON	C K JENNINGS	R J FOWLER
MISS E B KNAPMAN	P D M ROWLAND	J R TIMMS

Senior and Junior House Officers

G R STYLES	R B STILES	F M WARREN
G G DAVIS	L D G BROWN	A R HENWOOD
P J SHELDRICK	R J BROWNLEE	T C HUGHES
C R W BIRKETT	L K WALDEN	R S MARTIN
D BUCKLAND	N NICHOLAS	A F SMITH
D D C HAMILTON	J C FISHPOOL	L M LLOYD
J P B PENGELLY	G D PAMELY	MISS J GORDON-RALPH
A H CHIVERS	M BERNSTEIN	

Sister in Charge

MISS M G THOMPSON	SRN
MISS D M PARKER	SRN
MISS N W DAWES	SRN 1

1951-1960

Lecturers, Tutor and Recognised Teachers

L E CLAREMONT	H S M CRABB
H J DREW-SMYTHE	F R HOGBIN
W A JACKMANW	TREVOR JOHNSON
A 0 CHICK	E H EHRMANN

A R MACGREGOR
B N NEILSON
D VERO
J G J KEENE
P A WATLING
I W CAMERON
A J SEAR
D G LYON
D N NOBLE
C H VIGAR
MRS T BETCHERS
D A PEARCE
E J R MORGAN
J J MACKENNA
J B O'MAHONY

Senior Registrars and Registrars

E W B VARLEY
J A L IRWIN
J A L NELSON
MISS D M V CAMPBELL
M A BURLEY
A J DRINNAN
G E MOORE
G B SUMMERS GILL

Senior and Junior House Officers

G D EVERARD
A ROSENSTRAUGH
D BIRKHAHN
J D HOLGATE
M D PROSSER
I CAMERON
W B SENIOR
MISS SOBKIEWICZ
N DYER
W I MAKSYMIAK
MISS V H BREWER
K R TYRRELL
R J PRATT
MISS B ASTILL
W TELLERMAN
I L BUSBRIDGE
G D HOPKINS
I AFTER
P C SMITH
L D WALMSLEY
H C TAGG
J H CURTHOYS
J S P BRITTON
J A NOWELL
A D SCARBOROUGH
J O'NEILL
JAW TAYLOR
C CAMERON
B F MAHLE
S P CHATTERJEA
R J SMITH
N BAR
MISS J M COX
C W GOODMAN
W T G PHILIPPS
T A HYLAND
R S YOUNG

Sister in Charge

MISS N W DAWES	SRN
MISS K S DAVISON	SRN

APPENDIX 3

DENTAL HOSPITAL AND SCHOOL STAFF IN 1988

These appear as set out in Levers 1989; (* indicates a part-time appointment.)

A. CHILD DENTAL HEALTH

Professor
C D STEPHENS OBE; BDS; MDS; FDSRCS; M.Orth RCS (1984)

Consultant Senior Lecturer
P J M CRAWFORD BDS; MScD; FDSRCS

Lecturers
I A BALL LDS; FDSRCS; DDPHRCS (Paediatric Dentistry)
I D BROWN PhD; BDS; FDSRCS; D Orth RCS (Orthodontics)

Clinical Lecturers (ie those holding hospital contracts)
T B DOWELL MSc; BDS; LDSRCS; DDPHRCS* (Community Dentistry)
(The Regional & District Dental Officer)
N W T HARRADINE BDS; MB,BS; MSc; D Orth RCS, FDS* (Orthodontics)
I S HATHORN BDS; FDSRCS: D Orth RCS* (Orthodontics)
J C STEPHENSON BDS; FDSRCS: D Orth RCS* (Orthodontics)

Recognised Teachers
G DUGGAN BDS; DDPHRCS* (Paediatric Dentistry)
D K STABLES BDS; DDPHRCS* (Paediatric Dentistry)
MARION K STEPHENS BDS; LDSRCS* (Orthodontics)
G J TUCKER BDS; DDPHRCS* (Paediatric Dentistry)

Tutors
M RUTH EVANS BDS; MScD; D Orth RCS; FDSRCPS (Orthodontics)
KATHRYN M POSTLEWAITE BDS; MSc; FDSRCPS; D Orth RCS (Orthodontics)*

B. CONSERVATIVE DENTISTRY

Professor
R J ELDERTON PhD; BDS; LDSRCS (1985)

Consultant Senior Lecturer
C B G JENKINS PhD; BDS; MDS; LDS; FDSRCS

Lecturers

LOUISE V FOSTER BDS
G R HOOPER BDS*
SUSAN M HOOPER BDS
K J MARSHALL BDS
K ROBERTS BDS; FDSRCS; MGDSRCS*

Recognised Teachers

C J BELL BDS; MGDSRCS* (also in Prosthetics)
S P CHADWICK BDS*
D L CRAYTON BDS*
P G KEETON BDS*
J LUCIA BDS* (also in Prosthetics)
R C MILLER BDS* (also in Prosthetics)
LOUISE NASH BDS*
D C ROCKEY BDS*
I J STANDING BDS*
BAG TURNER BDS*

C. ORAL MEDICINE. SURGERY AND PATHOLOGY

Professor

C M SCULLY BSc; PhD;BDS;MB,BS;LDSRCS; FDSRCPS; FRCPath (1982)

Consultant Senior Lecturers

J W EVESON PhD; BDS; FDSRCPS; MRCPath (Oral Medicine and Pathology)
S S PRIME PhD; BDS; FDSRCPS (Oral Medicine)
J P SHEPHERD MSc; PhD; BDS; FDSRCS (Oral and Maxillofacial Surgery)
R G SMITH BChD; MDS; FDSRCS (Periodontology)
R W MATTHEWS PhD; BDS; MDS (Oral Medicine and Oral Surgery)

Lecturers

SARAH L MANTON PhD; BDS; FDSRCS (Oral Medicine and Oral Surgery)
ISABEL J CRANE BSc; PhD Wellcome Lecturer in Immunology

Clinical Lecturers

M J GRIFFITHS BDS; MB, BS; FDS RCS* (Oral Medicine and Oral Surgery)
G H IRVINE BDS; MB, ChB; FDSRCSE; FRCS* (Oral and Maxillofacial Surgery)
M J LUTTERLOCH BDS; MB, BS; FDSRCS* (Oral and Maxillofacial Surgery)
M MIDDA BDS; FDSRCS; FFRCSI* Periodontology)
G M PELL BDS; MB, BS; FDSRCS* (Oral and Maxillofacial Surgery)
J W ROSS LDS; FDSRCS* (Oral and Maxillofacial Surgery)
A H YOUNG BDS; FDSRCS; FDSRCSE; FFDRCSI* (Oral and Maxillofacial Surgery)

Special Lecturer
B G H LEVERS MSc; PhD

Recognised Teachers and Tutors
J GREENMAN BSc; PhD* (Oral Microbiology)
A F V FITTER BDS; DDPHRCS* (Oral Medicine and Oral Surgery)
G M JONES BDS; MB, BS; FDSRCPS* (Oral Medicine and Oral Surgery)

Research Staff (MRC Dental Unit)
D F G POOLE BSc; PhD* (Research Fellow in Oral Medicine)
KAREN M PORTER BDS* (Research Fellow in Oral Medicine & Oral Surgery)
SALLY V R NIXON BDS; FDS; LDS* (Research Fellow in Oral Medicine & Oral Surgery)
S R FLINT BDS; MB, BS; FDSRCS (Research Associate in Oral Medicine)
L GATHERCOLE MSc; PhD (Research Associate in Oral Medicine & Oral Surgery)
G H DIBDIN MSc; PhD* (Research Associate in Oral Medicine)
S R PORTER BSc; PhD; BDS; FDSRCS* (Research Associate in Oral Medicine)
P SHELLIS MSc; PhD* (Research Associate in Oral Medicine)
J E TYLER MSc; PhD* (Research Associate in Oral Medicine)
S M GAME BSc; PhD (Research Assistant in Oral Medicine)
S MUTLU DDS; MSc (Research Assistant in Oral Medicine)
MARY J DONNELLY
LOUISE K TORRANCE

D. PROSTHETIC DENTISTRY AND DENTAL CARE OF THE ELDERLY

Professor
A HARRISON TD; PhD; BDS; FDSRCS (1987)

Lecturers
A C WATKINSON BChD; MDS; FDSRCSE; DRDRCSE
D R WILLIAMS BSc; BDS

Special Lecturer
K R COWLES LDS*

Clinical Lecturer
C M WOODHEAD BDS; MSc; FDSRCSE*

Recognised Teacher
P N JONES BDS*
S J MARSH-SMITH BDS*
P MILLER BDS; LDS; DDPH*
N J NEWTON BDS* \
J D SCARRATT BDS; DDPH*

YVONNE L M THOMAS BDS*
RUTH COLLIS BDS
J HINDLE BDS

E. TECHNICAL STAFF

Chief Instructor

R HUGGETT MSc; CGIA; FBIST; FETC

Deputy Chief Instructor

G BIDDLECOMBE FETC

Instructors

R GARN FETC
A D TELFORD FETC
C C WRIGHT FETC

F. Sister in Charge

MRS Y THEYER SRN

APPENDIX 4

DENTAL HOSPITAL AND SCHOOL STAFF IN 2011

HOSPITAL STAFF

It had been intended to include in our centenary year the names of current dental staff to provide a comparison with earlier surveys but this is now thought to be inappropriate. Not only has the undergraduate intake of the School increased by 40% since 1988 when Levers carried the last survey, but there have been fundamental changes since then in the structure of the profession which makes any comparison misleading. First there has been the introduction by the General Dental Council of dental specialist lists. Thus in addition to consultants and associate specialists, the Hospital now has fully trained and registered dental specialists. UK compliance with European Directives has meant that our 19 registrar posts, like all others in the UK, are full time training posts and senior registrars no longer exist. House Officer appointments have been replaced by the first Vocational Training year, shortly to become Dental Foundation Year 1. Senior House Officer posts, which still exist, will then be absorbed into Dental Foundation Year 2. Secondly the establishment of professions complementary to dentistry by the GDC means we now have a large Dental Care Professional School (nurses, hygienist, and therapists) with a staff of 14 tutors.

On the face of it the Dental Hospital now has an NHS staff of 384 but this includes staff of the DCP School, officers of the Community Dental Service and managerial, secretarial, clerical and support staff which have not been included in previous analyses. Many of these staff are part time or are shared with other hospitals and clinics.

UNIVERSITY STAFF

There are similar difficulties when attempting to compare current dental academic staffing with earlier assessments as there are no longer identifiable departments. Also in 1988 the Medical Research Council's Dental Unit closed with loss of its valuable research staff but the continuing pressure on universities to undertake outstanding research remained. This has lead to a distinction being made in the School between " teaching" and "research staff" Many of the latter are full time non -clinical staff some of whom are funded on short term research grants.

What might otherwise have lead to a reduction in clinical academic staff in the School has been offset partly by the additional fee income arising from the increased undergraduate and postgraduate dental intake and partly through the use of computer based learning.

University paid Dental School Staff 2011

Professors

Jenkinson	Howard	Professor of Oral Microbiology
West	Nicola	Professor in Restorative Dentistry
Kilpatrick	Nicola	Professor in Paediatric Dentistry
Ness	Andy	Professor of Epidemiology
O'Sullivan	Dominic	Professor in Restorative Dentistry
Prime	Stephen	Professor of Experimental Pathology
Sandy	Jonathan	Professor of Orthodontics
Scully	Crispian	Professor in Oral Medicine
Thomas	Steve	Professor In Oral and Maxillofacial Surgery

Readers

Ireland	Anthony	Reader in Orthodontics
Middleton	Jim	Reader in Cellular Immunology
Robb	Nigel	Reader in Restorative Dentistry
Su	Bo	Reader in Biomaterials

Senior Lecturers

Barbour	Michele	Senior Lecturer in Dental Materials Science and Biomaterials
Crawford	Peter	Consultant Senior Lecturer in Paediatric Dentistry
Dymock	David	Senior Lecturer in Oral Microbiology
Drugan	Caroline	Consultant Senior Lecturer in Dental Public Health
Gray	Gordon	Senior Lecturer in Restorative Dentistry (Conservative Dentistry)
Hooper	Susan	Consultant Senior Lecturer Restorative Dentistry (Conservative Dentistry)
Jagger	Robert	Consultant Senior Lecturer in Restorative Dentistry
Leary	Sam	Senior Lecturer in Statistics
Pring	Miranda	Consultant Senior Lecturer in Oral Maxillofacial Pathology

Lecturers

Atkinson	Charlotte	Lecturer in Nutrition, Epidemiology & Population Oral Health Research
Blum	Igor	Lecturer in Restorative Dentistry
Fleming	Carla	Lecturer in Oral Surgery
Ke	Melissa	Lecturer in Health Economics
Main	Barry	Lecturer in Oral and Maxillofacial Surgery
Nobbs	Angela	Lecturer in Oral Microbiology
Waylen	Andrea	Lecturer in Psychology

Clinical Lecturers

Cirillo	Nicola	Clinical Lecturer

GDP/Clinical Teachers/Teaching Fellows

Adams	Alison	GDP / Clinical Teacher
Al-Qudah	Aladdin	Clinical Teacher
Beevers	Daniel	GDP / Clinical Teacher in Oral Surgery
Bhatt	Reena	Clinical Teaching Fellow in Paediatric Dentistry
Boswell	Gillian	Clinical Teaching Fellow in Restorative Dentistry
Brown	Katie	GDP /Clinical Teacher
Daud	Alaa	Clinical Skills Teacher
Fullaway	Carl	Clinical Teacher in Restorative Dentistry
Green	Joseph	Teaching Fellow
Hague	Angela	Senior Teaching Fellow
Harris	Timothy	GDP / Clinical Teacher in Oral Surgery
Mallinson	Julie	Clinical Teacher in Restorative Dentistry
Marsden	Lucy	Teaching Fellow in Paediatric Dentistry
Nash	Louise	Clinical Lead - Community Based Teaching
Rooney	Jane	Clinical Teaching Fellow
Sellen	Carole	Teaching Fellow in Dental Technology
Sellen	Philip	Teaching Fellow in Dental Technology
Waller	Lynne	Clinical Teacher
Woolerton	Gill	General Dental Practitioner/Clinical Teacher

Dental Tutors

Chapman	Alison	Dental Hygiene
Harwood	Alison	Dental Hygiene/Dental Therapy
Whitley	Sarah	Dental Hygiene

Research Staff

Brittan	Jane	Research Technician
Claydon	Nicholas	Clinical Research Fellow in Prosthodontics & Periodontology
Davies	Maria	Clinical Research Manager
Dutton	Lindsay	Research Technician
Jones	Sian	Research Associate
Seong	Joon	Clinical Research Fellow
Sharif	Nusret	Research Technician
Sjostrom	Terje	Research Assistant
Soro	Valeria	Research Technician
Sprague	Susan	Research Technician
Wintle	Zoe	Dental Nurse (Research)

Technical Staff

McGlynn	Michael	Head of Dental Production Laboratories

Cresswell	Wendy	Senior Chief Prosthetics Dental Technician
Edge	Rob	Senior Chief Orthodontic Technician
Sealey	John	Senior Chief Dental Technician
Wedekind	Michael	Chief Dental Technician
Rigby	Mark	Chief Dental Technician
Leggett	Victoria	Chief Orthodontic Technician
Bessant	Michelle	Senior Dental Technician
Bisp	Richard	Senior Dental Technician
Blackaby	Caroline	Senior Dental Technician
Easterling	Marcus	Senior Dental Technician
Foxall-Giess	Mark	Senior Dental Technician
Georgiou	Tracy	Senior Dental Technician
Herborn	Nicholas	Senior Dental Technician
Hogg	Jerry	Senior Dental Technician
Horne	Theresa	Senior Dental Technician
Leggett	Gregor	Senior Dental Technician
McGrath	Mark	Senior Dental Technician
Perry	Alan	Senior Dental Technician
Rowbern	Marta	Senior Dental Technician
Thorne	Emma	Senior Dental Technician
Tyacke	Jennifer	Senior Dental Technician
Webb	Andrea	Senior Dental Technician
West	Nicola	Senior Dental Technician/ Maxillo Facial Technician
Tsiopani	Lucy	Dental Technician
Woodland	Craig	Dental Technician

Administrative Staff

Cooper	Faye	Executive Assistant
Nunn	Nunn	School Administrator
Milne-Day	Laura	Academic Administrator

APPENDIX 5

THE MANAGEMENT OF THE DENTAL HOSPITAL AND SCHOOL

Initially the part time lecturers in dental anatomy, dental mechanics, dental surgery and dental metallurgy came under the authority of the Professor of Physiology. One presumes that when the Medical School became incorporated into the University College, he reported to the Faculty Board on dental matters.

The University gained its Charter in 1909 and by 1911 there were minutes of the Medical Board which referred to a Dental Subcommittee.[196] From then on regular reports were received from it. By 1913 W.R.Ackland was noted in the Medical Board minutes as being reappointed as one of the "Lecturers in charge of Departments" and this annual reappointment seems to have continued until his resignation in April 1923 at which point LE Claremont took over until his resignation in 1929.

In 1934 PJ Stoy was appointed as the first full time lecturer in a dental subject (dental mechanics). It is not clear what his management role was but since he was the only full time lecturer it must have been to him that the Dean of Faculty would have turned on dental matters. By January 1940 Stoy's position as Dental Assistant Dean had been confirmed.

When the Dental Hospital opened in 1939 a Management Committee was established. This first met 4th on December of that year. It was responsible to the University Council and contained a representative elected by the honorary dental surgeons as well as the Medical Officer of Health for the City. There was also a dental house committee chaired by the Assistant Dean Philip Stoy which reported to the Management Committee. Stoy also reported on academic matters to the Board of Faculty of which he was a member.

In the late 1940s in the run up to the start of the National Health Service the Vice Chancellor Sir Philip Morris, an ex officio member of the Management Committee, took the chair. Arthur Darling attended the first meeting of the committee on 30th October 1947 and at the next meeting Philip Stoy's departure to the Chair in Belfast was announced. John Snawdon who had qualified in Bristol in 1935 now took over as Dental Assistant Dean. Both the Dental Assistant Dean and the new Professor of Dental Surgery sat on the Faculty Board .

With its incorporation in to the National Health Service the Dental Hospital administration now had a dual structure. What had been a Management Committee reporting the University Council became a Joint Management Committee chaired by the Vice Chancellor Sir Philip Morris. This reported both to the University and to the Board of Governors of the United Bristol Hospitals. The new Joint Management Committee received reports from the Dental Sub Committee of the University Faculty Board. The Dental House Committee ultimately became the Dental Division of the District Health Authority in the NHS Reorganisation of 1973.

Perhaps as a result of necessary administrative restructuring after John Snawdon's death the Board of Dental Studies came into being in 1958/9 as the successor to the Dental Subcommittee of the Board of Faculty. Its Standing Orders were approved at the meeting of Faculty Board on the 10th January 1958. They were

1. The Board of Dental studies shall meet at least once in each academic term and at such other times as the board itself may decide.
2. The Board shall regulate and direct dental studies and examinations subject to review by the Board of the Faculty Medicine and provided in the statutes of the University and shall accordingly submit reports to the Medical Board.
3. The Board shall appoint its own Chairman who shall be elected annually from the members of the Board at its last regular meeting in the summer term and shall take office at the beginning of the following academic year.
4. Except as otherwise provided in the case of representatives appointed by outside bodies the members shall be appointed by Senate on the recommendation of the Medical Board and such members as are not appointed ex officio shall be subject to annual re-appointment without limitation of term.
5. The board shall regulate its own procedure provided only that the conduct of its business shall be in accord with common University practice.
6. The Registrar shall act as secretary of the Board.

Arthur Darling became the Board's first Chairman, a post he retained until the session 1973/4. Professor Bradford took over as Dental Assistant Dean until the session 1969/70. By this time there was also a Dental Preclinical Dean, an office held shortly after his arrival by Prof Declan Anderson. Thereafter each of these appointments as Dean rotated among the non-professorial staff and tended to be held for a term of three years.

From the time of his appointment in 1948 until his retirement in 1982 Arthur Darling retained the title of Director of Dental Studies at which point the title lapsed. For a period of three years the Chairman of the Board of Dental Studies acted as Head of School at which point the latter was established. In November 1985 the key posts of Head of School and Clinical Dental Dean were redefined as follows:

HEAD OF THE CLINICAL DENTAL SCHOOL

PURPOSE

To undertake those external administrative appointments to which a University Dental representative is required.

ELIGIBILITY

A Clinical Dental Professor, the order of succession normally being that of seniority.

RESPONSIBILITIES

1. To represent the School on the following:

a) General Dental Council
b) Dental Education Advisory Council.
c) Regional Liaison Committee.
d) Avon District Liaison Committee
e) Association of Dental Deans in Europe.
f) Association of University Teaching Hospitals.

2. Be an ex officio member of the following:

a) Regional Postgraduate Dental Committee.
b) Regional Dental Committee.
c) Dental Specialist Sub Committee of the Regional Medical Committee.
d) Board of Medical Studies.

3. To convene and chair the informal meetings Heads of Clinical Dental Departments.

4. To ensure good maintenance of School Records in particular:

a) Plans of the Buildings and minutes and reports relating to the:

Scheduling and Building Committee.

b) reports of UGC and GDC visitation.
c) Such other reports as the Board of Studies shall agree or the Head of School feel appropriate.

5. To keep the Board of Dental Studies informed by a regular report to Board Meetings.

6. To keep the Dental Clinical Dean informed about matters which fall within his field of responsibility.

PERIOD OF OFFICE

Four years renewable for a further two.

APPOINTMENT

By Senate on the recommendation of the Board of Studies.

DUTIES OF DENTAL CLINICAL DEAN

1. To be responsible for the general welfare of undergraduate clinical dental students and to be regularly and readily accessible to students.
2. To be responsible for student discipline and to keep a record of any action taken in disciplining students.
3. To be responsible for authorising students' leave of absence, subject to the approval of senior University staff supervisors in the clinical departments.
4. To be Chairman of the following sub-committees of the Board of Dental Studies :-
   i) Dental Clinical Students Progress Committee
   ii) Dental Clinical Students Curriculum Committee
   iii) Dental Clinical Students Staff/Student Liaison Committee
   iv) Human Disease Committee
5. As Chairman of the Clinical Dental Students' Progress Committee, to maintain records of students academic progress, to record any action taken in encouraging improved performances, and to inform the student's personal tutor of such action.
6. As Chairman of the Clinical Dental Students Curriculum Committee, to be responsible for the day to day running of the undergraduate clinical course.
7. As Chairman of the Staff/Student Liaison Committee, to be responsible for maintaining good staff/student relationships.
8. As Chairman of the Human Disease Committee, to liaise closely with the Human Disease Course co-ordinator in administering the course.
9. To be a member of the Admissions Committee, the Building & Scheduling Committee and the Health & Safety Committee.
10. To be responsible for the clinical dental students' Personal Tutor Scheme, informing tutors about students who may require help in academic or personal matters.
11. To be responsible for administering the clinical part of the Final BDS Examination in consultation with the Heads of Departments. To maintain the mark sheets for the whole examination, to chair the final examination meeting and to send the mark sheet, signed by the examiners, to the University Examinations office, and to post the pass list on the Dental School board after the results have been approved.
12. To organise the General Dental Council's Statutory Examination when the Council requests, and the Board of Dental Studies agree, that the examination should be arranged in Bristol.
13. To co-ordinate the senior students' electives.
14. To make arrangements for undergraduate students visiting Bristol from other dental

schools.

15. To make arrangements for prospective dental students to visit the Dental School.
16. To be Chairman of the Link with Hannover Committee, co-ordinating plans either for visiting Hannover (liaising with the responsible person at the Hannover Dental School) or for entertaining visitors from Hannover.
17. To keep a record of applications from postgraduate students wishing to pursue studies here, and to pass these applications on to the appropriate Head of Department.
18. To organise Prize Giving and other semi-formal functions.
19. To keep the Head of the School and the Board of Dental Studies informed about matters which fall within their fields of responsibility.

These duties may be altered only by agreement of the Board of Dental Studies.

PERIOD OF OFFICE

By annual re-appointment for normally not more than 5 years.

APPOINTMENT

By the Board of Faculty on the recommendation of the Board of Dental Studies.

This structure remained largely unchanged until the major review of the School's structure in 2008 referred to in Chapter 10.

APPENDIX 6

HOLDERS OF KEY ACADEMIC APPOINTMENTS 1967-2011

	Head of School	Dental Clinical Dean	Chairman of Board of Dental Studies	Chairman of Dental Education Committee
1967/8		Professor Bradford	Professor Darling	
1968/9		Professor Bradford	Professor Darling	
1969/70		Professor Berry	Professor Darling	
1970/1		Professor Berry	Professor Darling	
1971/2		Professor Berry	Professor Darling	
1972/3		Jim Fletcher	Professor Darling	
1973/4		Jim Fletcher	Graham Charlton	
1974/5		Jim Fletcher	Graham Charlton	
1975/6		Graham Charlton	Graham Charlton	
1976/7		Graham Charlton	Jim Fletcher	
1977/8		Graham Charlton	Jim Fletcher	
1978/9		Abdul Adatia	Jim Fletcher	
1979/80		Abdul Adatia	Graham Charlton	
1980/1		Abdul Adatia	Graham Charlton	
1981/2		Dr Reg Andlaw	Graham Charlton	
1982/3	NONE	Dr Reg Andlaw	Professor Stephens	
1983/4	NONE	Dr Reg Andlaw	Professor Stephens	
1984/5	NONE	Dr Reg Andlaw	Professor Stephens	
1985/6	NONE	Dr Reg Andlaw	Professor Stephens	
1986/7	Informal[197]	Dr Reg Andlaw	Dr Clive Jenkins	
1986/8	Professor Skully[198]	Robin Matthews	Dr Clive Jenkins	
1988/9	Professor Scully	Robin Matthews	Dr Clive Jenkins	
1989/0	Professor Scully	Robin Matthews	Prof Harrison	
1990/1	Professor Scully	Robin Matthews	Prof Harrison	
1991/2	Professor Scully	Robin Matthews	Prof Harrison	
1992/3	Professor Scully	Ken Marshall	Prof Harrison	
1993/4	Prof Harrison	Ken Marshall	Head of School	
1994/5	Prof Harrison	Ken Marshall	Head of School	
1995/6	Prof Harrison	Ken Marshall	Head of School	
1996/7	Prof Harrison	Ken Marshall	Head of School	
1997/8	Prof Harrison	Ken Marshall	Head of School	
1999/0	Prof Harrison	Ken Marshall	Head of School	
2000/1	Prof Harrison	Ken Marshall	Head of School	Prof Sandy
2001/2	Prof Cowpe	Gordon Gray	Head of School	Prof Sandy
2002/3	Prof Cowpe	Gordon Gray	Head of School	Prof Sandy
2003/4	Prof Cowpe	Gordon Gray	Head of School	Prof Sandy
2004/5	Prof Steve Prime	Gordon Gray	Head of School	Prof Cowpe
2005/6	Prof Steve Prime	Gordon Gray	Head of School	Prof Cowpe
2006/7	Prof Steve Prime	Gordon Gray	Head of School	Prof Cowpe
2007/8	Prof Sandy	Gordon Gray	Head of School	Dr D Dymock
2008/9	Prof Sandy	Gordon Gray	Head of School	Daryll Jagger
2009/10	Prof Sandy	Gordon Gray	Head of School	Peter Crawford

Dental Postgraduate Dean

Prof David Berry	March 1984 - April 1987
Derek Seel	May 1987 - December 1991
Alastair Miller	January 1992 -

BIBLIOGRAPHY

British Dental Association. The advance of the dental profession. British Dental Association. London, 1979.

Carlton D. A University for Bristol. Bristol University Press. Bristol, 1984.

Jerrard J. Reminiscences. University of Bristol Womens Club. Bristol, 1997.

Levers BGH. A history of the Bristol Dental School and Hospital. University of Bristol. Bristol, 1989.

Perry CB. The Bristol Medical School. The Bristol Branch of the Historical Society, Bristol, 1964.

Saunders CJG. The University of Bristol Dental School and Hospital. The Board of Governors of the United Bristol Hospitals. Bristol, 1964.

Saunders CJG. The United Bristol Hospitals. The United Bristol Hospitals. Bristol,1965.

Seward M. Open Wide: Memoir of the Dental Dame. The Memoir Club. Durham, 2009.

Smith GM. A history of the Bristol Royal Infirmary. J W Arrowsmith Ltd. Bristol, 1917.

Watson S. Secret Underground Bristol. Bristol Junior Chambers. Bristol, 1991.

REFERENCES

1. Jackson R Archaeological excavations at Upper Maudlin Street in 1973, 1976 and 1999. Bristol and Avon Archaeology 2000 17: 92-95.
2. Ponsford MW. Excavations at Greyfriars Bristol. City of Bristol Museum and Art Gallery. Bristo1. 1975.
3. Weare GE: Collectanea Relating to the Friars Minor of Bristol, W. Bennett. Bristo1, 1893.
4. Little B. The Story of Bristol. The Redcliffe Press, Bristol 1991. Page 27.
5. Watson S. Secret Underground Bristol. Bristol Junior Chamber. Bristol, 1991. Pages 104-119.
6. Weare GE. A collectanea relating to the Bristol Friars Minor (Gray Friars) and their Convent. W. Bennet, Bristo1,1893. Page 47.
7. Weare GE. A collectanea relating to the Bristol Friars Minor (Gray Friars) and their Convent. W. Bennet, Bristol, 1893. Page 33-36.
8. Williams B. The Infirmary Burial Ground..Report for the Charitable Trusts of the Bristol Royal Infirmary, Bristol, 2003.
9. Moravian Church Diary 1804-1806 Central Library Bristol. Local History ref 26605.
10. Dresser M. Sisters and brethren: power propriety and gender among the Bristol Moravians 1746-1833. Social History 21: 304-329.
11. This was presumably the mediaeval use of the word meaning " company".
12. Dresser M In Historic churches and church life in Bristol. Joseph Bettey (ed) Bristol and Gloucestershire Archaeological Society. Bristol 2001 page 137.
13. Whaley B. John Smith and Sons of Bristol :Worklist. British Institute of Organ Studies Reporter 1999, 23 (4) http://www.npor.org.uk/Reporter/oct99/e1099.htm
14. See http://www.badham.org.uk/badham/B1NS_newsletter%20examples/NL_5-3.html
15. Pigot's Directory of Gloucestershire 1830.
16. Saunders CJG The United Bristol Hospitals. Part 2 Chapter 4. United Bristol Hospitals. Bristol, 1965.
17. 'Waifs and Wanderers in St Jude's', in The Homes of the Bristol Poor. William Lewis & Sons, Bristol.1884 (reprinted from the Bristol Mercury),
18. Records of St. John's Diocesan Home, and of its predecessors. Bristol Record Office.
19. Wright, Mary & Mellor, Penny. Kingsdown: Bristol's Vertical Suburb Phillimore, Bristol, 2009.
20. Central Reference Library Bristol. Booklet reference M0005714AN.
21. See McAuley JE Med Hist. 1970 October; 14: 418–419.
22. Hillam C Professional Education for dentistry before 1859. Br Dent J 1987 163: 204-207.
23. Woodhouse AJ. Address to the British Dental Association. Journal of the British Dental Association 1897 18: 21-31.
24. Smith GM. A history of the Bristol Royal Infirmary. J W Arrowsmith Ltd., Bristol. 1917. Page 366.
25. Charles Gaines, one of the first three medical students to take the conjoint examination had been appointed as Surgeon Dentist in Bath as early as1861.
26. Smith GM. A history of the Bristol Royal Infirmary. J W Arrowsmith Ltd., Bristol. 1917. Page 392.
27. Spencer EM Notes on the history of dental dispensaries. Medical History 1982, 26: 47-66.
28. British Dental Association. The advance of the dental profession. British Dental Association, London, 1979. Page 66.
29. Notice of removal, Bristol Times and Mirror, 4th January 1897.
30. Smith GM. A history of the Bristol Royal Infirmary. J W Arrowsmith Ltd., Bristol. 1917. Page 360.
31. British Dental Association. The Advance of the Dental Profession. BDA. London, 1979. Page 2.
32. British Dental Association. The Advance of the Dental Profession. BDA. London, 1979. Pages 3-11.
33. These were bound as part of the University College Calendar until it became the entry for the Medical Faculty of the College in 1893/4.
34. Perry CB The Bristol Medical School. The Bristol Branch of the Historical Society 1964. Page 15.
35. University College Calendar Session 1899 –1900. Page 178.
36. University College Calendar Session 1899 –1900. Page 208.

37. Smith TM. A History of the Bristol Royal Infirmary. J.W.Arrowsmith, Bristol 1917. Page 392.
38. Perry C B. The Bristol Medical School. The Bristol Branch of the Historical Association. Bristol, 1984. Page 19.
39. University College Calendar Session 1906 –1907. Page 251.
40. Stoy P The Bristol Dental School 1874-1940. British Dental Journal 1947, 82: 141.
41. Stoy P The Bristol Dental School 1874-1940. British Dental Journal 1947, 82: 142.
42. This was the Rt Hon (Sir) Francis Dyke Acland, no relation the William Robert Ackland.
43. The same year as W G Grace entered the Bristol Medical School!
44. Notice of removal, Bristol Times and Mirror, 4th January 1897.
45. Cunningham G. British Dental Journal 1891 12: 244.
46. Report of the Dean Minute 3 of the Board of the Faculty of Medicine 26th September 1913, University of Bristol.
47. Medical Faculty Board Minutes 15th January1915. Minute 3.
48. Medical Faculty Board Minutes 30th April 1915. Minute 5.
49. By 1938 there were 5400 such "Approved Societies" nationally offering dental treatment as an additional benefit to a membership of 13,070,000. See Ross R. Dentistry in the 1930s. Dental History Magazine 2009, 3:13-17.
50. Medical Faculty Board Minutes 28th February 1919. Minute 9.
51. Medical Faculty Board Minutes 26th November 1920. Minute 7.
52. Medical Faculty Board Minutes 16th November 1918. Minute 1.
53. Medical Faculty Board Minutes 26th November 1920. Minute 6.
54. Medical Faculty Board Minutes 18th November 1920. Minute 3.
55. Medical Faculty Board Minutes 22nd February 1922. Minute 4.
56. Medical Faculty Board Minutes 19th January 1923. Minute 4.
57. Medical Faculty Board Minutes 23rd November 1923 Minute 5.
58. Medical Faculty Board Minutes 18th June 1926. Minute 2c.
59. Medical Faculty Board Minutes 2nd March 1928. Minute 9.
60. Medical Faculty Board Minute 9th October 1928 Minute 6.
61. Medical Faculty Board Minutes 7th June 1929. Minute 6.
62. Medical Faculty Board Minutes4th October 1929. Minute 7, 8.
63. Levers BGH.A history of the Bristol Dental School and Hospital. University of Bristol 1989, Chapter 3..
64. Medical Faculty Board Minutes 31st May 1935. Minute 7.
65. Leighton BC The Dental Education Advisory Council: 50 years. British Dental Journal 1980 149: 267-268.
66. Burke P. Personal Communication, April 2011.
67. University of Bristol Dental Management Committee Minutes. 15th January 1940. Minute 6.
68. University of Bristol Dental Management Committee Minutes. 17th May 1940. Minute 6.
69. University of Bristol Dental Management Committee Minutes 19th June 1940. Minute 2.
70. On the night of 24th November 1940 the centre of Bristol suffered heavy bombing raids, and the Prince's Theatre, along with the Coliseum were totally destroyed. The BBC transferred many of its departments to Bristol, as London was taking the brunt of the Blitz. The popular wartime radio programme "ITMA" (It's That Man Again") starring Tommy Handley was broadcast from Clifton Parish Hall in Bristol throughout this period. See http://www.its-behind-you.com/princesbristol.html
71. Bristol was the fifth most heavily bombed city in Britain. On the 2nd November 1940 a severe bombing raid destroyed or damaged over 10,000 houses, with much loss of life.
72. This was a time when the St Johns conduits built by Carmelite Friars in 1267 again came into their own and at one time during the blitz the St John's Fountain on the wall of St Johns at the Wall in Nelson Street was the only source of drinking water. The cisterns along it length were used by fire fighters to douse fires on Park Street (see Watson S. Secret Underground Bristol. Bristol Junior Chambers,1991. Pages 112-3.)
73. Official figures were 156 killed, 149 seriously injured,121 slightly injured..
74. Marmion V. The Bristol Eye Hospital – celebrating 200 years of service. The Bristol Medico Historial Society, Bristol 2010. Page 53.
75. Smith E, Cottell B. A History of the Royal Dental Hospital of London 1858-1985 The Athlone Press, London, 1997. Page 42.

76. Transactions of the Odontological Society Volume II Cox and Wyman, London, 1861. Pages 107-109.
77. Saunders CJG. The University of Bristol Dental School and Hospital The Board of Governors of the United Bristol Hospitals, Bristol, 1964. Page 66.
78. Stoy P The Bristol Dental School 1874-1940.Br Dent J 1947 82: 142.
79. Saunders CJG. The University of Bristol Dental School and Hospital The Board of Governors of the United Bristol Hospitals, Bristol, 1964. Page 15.
80. Stoy P The Bristol Dental School 1874-1940.Br Dent J 1947 82: 142.
81. Stoy P.J. Personal communication January 1996.
82. Ibid.
83. University of Bristol Dental Management Committee Minutes 11th February 1943 Minute 4.
84. University of Bristol Dental Management Committee Minutes.27th May 1948 Minute 7.
85. University of Bristol Dental Management Committee Minutes 31st January 1946 Minute 6.
86. University of Bristol Dental Management Committee Minutes. 30th January1947 Minute 5.
87. University of Bristol Dental Management Committee Minutes. 31st October 1946. Minute 6.
88. University of Bristol Dental Management Committee Minutes 29th January 1948. Minute 8.
89. Patricia Burke (BDS Ubrist.,1942) Personal communication July 2011.
90. Obituary British Dental Journal 1988,164: 129.
91. Saunders CJG. The University of Bristol Dental Hospital and School. Board of Governors of the United Bristol Hospitals, Bristol,1964. Page 22.
92. Woods A R. The Western Counties Branch of the British Dental Association, Bristol, 1958.
93. Minutes of the joint Management Committee of the Dental Hospital 4th November 1948 Minute 11..
94. Minutes of the joint Management Committee of the Dental Hospital 16th October 1950 Minute 3.
95. Minutes of the joint Management Committee of the Dental Hospital 21st July 1953 Minute 8.
96. Obituary, British Spelaeological Society 1978 See www.ubss.org.uk/resourc/roceedings/vol15/UBSS_Proc_15_1_3-5.pdf
97. University of Bristol Dental Management Committee Minutes 29th May 1947. Minute 2.
98. University of Bristol Minutes of the Dental Hospital Extension Equipment Sub Committee 11th February 1963.
99. Face to Face with Declan Anderson. Dental Practice 1992, 30: (23) 1-2.
100. Minutes of the University Scheduling and Building Subcommittee for the Dental Hospital, 6th February 1970.
101. Fletcher JP, Hobbs K, Hunt AC, Knapp MS, Linton AH, McCarthy CF. Bristol human disease course for dental students. British Journal of Medical Education 1967,1: 381-385.
102. A request made by me to Professor Darling that he stand down after 30 years as "Director of Dental Studies" and let there be an elected head, as in all other dental schools, met with a flat refusal and the comment that " there is no one I can trust to run my school". Chris Stephens,2011.
103. This is the reason why the present Queen Elizabeth Building is still often referred to by retired members of staff as the Phase I building.
104. Letter from Charles Clarke to R Northcott.28th April 1975.
105. Geddes D. Burnt out dons fading away on full pay. The Times 2nd October 1981.
106. In December 1985 Sir Keith Joseph announced legislation for abolishing tenure.
107. Darling AI. Teaching and research the University's role. Contact Point. 1979 10 (2): 11-12.
108. Obituary, John Hamilton Farrell . British Dental Journal 1981,150: 292.
109. Sheiham. A. Future patterns of dental care--manpower implications for industrialised countries. Br Dent J. 1989;167:51.
110. T Lehner T, Russell MW, Caldwell J, Smith R .Immunization with purified protein antigens from Streptococcus mutans against dental caries in rhesus monkeys. Infect Immun. 1981, 34: 407–415.
111. Letter from Professor Darling to the University Bursar Frank Ott. 4th November 1974.
112. Letter from Professor Crispian Scully to Professor Ian Silver 10th April 1989.
113. Medical Research Council Annual Report. British Dental Journal 1983, 154: 7.
114. In 1988/9 the UFC allocated £1,398,000 to the University for Clinical Dentistry only £966,000 of which was devolved to the School. Letter from Dean of the Faculty to Professor Scully 19/11/1990.

115. Minutes of the Meeting of the UFC and the University of Bristol to consider the effect of the NHS reforms 21st February 1991.
116. Newsletter. Volume 15 No 2 October 4th. University of Bristol, 1984.
117. The University Hospitals Association. A survey of the effects of reduced funding of Universities on Dental Schools and the NHS in England and Wales for the Academic Years 1984-1986 including references to the Academic Years 1981-1984. UHA, March 1987.
118. Report to the Nuffield Foundation. An inquiry into dental education. The Nuffield Foundation. London, 1980.
119. Report of the Dental Strategy Review Group. Towards better dental health- guidelines for the future. Department of Health and Social Security, London 1981
120. General Dental Council Recommendations concerning the Dental Curriculum. General Dental Council London, 1986.
121. Second Report of the Manpower Sub-Committee of the British Dental Association. British Dental Journal 1986 :161 (Suppl).
122. Report of the Committee of Enquiry into Unnecessary Dental Treatment. Department of Health and Social Security, London, 1986.
123. Phillimore AJ. University research performance indicators in practice: The University Grants Committee's evaluation of British universities, 1985–86. Research Policy 1998 18: 255-271.
124. Gillett R Serious anomalies in the UGC comparative evaluation of the research performance of psychology departments. Bulletin of the Psychological Society 1987, 40: 42-49.
125. This did call into question what "average" was in the exercise!
126. Elderton RJ. Scope for change in clinical practice. Journal of the Royal Society of Medicine 1985, 78: Supplement 7.
127. Anderson RJ. The changes in dental caries experience of 12-year-old school children in two Somerset schools. A review after an interval of 19 years. British Dental Journal 1984, 157:20-22.
128. Charles Clarke retired the following year on the occasion of which he received an Honorary Doctorate of Letters from the University.
129. Second Report of the Manpower Sub-Committee of the Council of the British Dental Association. Annex 2,pages 23-8, Proceedings of the Representative Board,14.6.86. Br Dent J1986;161 (Suppl)
130. Arthur Darling died on December 22nd 1987..
131. Naylor MN. One hundred years of dental education at Guys. The United Medical and Dental Schools of Guy's and St Thomas' Hospitals. London,1989. Page 79.
132. Fair exchange of academic robbery.The Independent. 2nd March 1989.
133. Doubling fees to increase competition. The Times Higher Education Supplement. April 14th 1989.
134. Committee on Higher Education (1963). The Robbins Report CMND 2154, paragraph 555.
135. Scully C. Letter to Professor A Harrison, 20th March1989.
136. Stephens CD. Letter to Professor RD Chambers.17th April 1989.
137. Scully C. Letter to Academic Staff 2nd July 1990.
138. Strictly an additional University representative for those Authorities which provided clinical facilities for a dental school as well as a medical school. This was always taken to mean a dental academic.
139. Vice-Chancellor's speech to Court. University Newsletter,1991, 21(8) :7.
140. News from the UFC. University Newsletter 1992 Vol 22 (11) 5th March 1992.
141. Decay of the Dentist. Leading Article. The Times, March 25th 1992..
142. Department of Health. Hospital Doctors: training for the future. The Report of the Working Group on Specialist Medical Training. (The Calman Report) Department of Health, London, 1993.
143. "Research quality that equates to attainable levels of national excellence in a majority of subject areas, or to international level in some"
144. Computers in Teaching Initiative in Clinical Medicine based at Bristol.
145. Nuffield Inquiry into the Education and training of personnel auxiliary to dentistry. The Nuffield Foundation, Oxford 1993.
146. Dentists Act 1984: 45 (1).
147. It had been rumoured since the end of March that he had been appointed Dean of the Eastman Dental Institute.
148. Supervised Training Group. Statement on Vocational Training May 1983.

149. Gainsford I. Dental Education : implementing the continuum. Journal of the Royal College of Surgeons of Edinburgh 1999, 44:141-145.
150. Anderssohn et al. The Joint Response of the British Orthodontic Societies to the Nuffield Inquiry into Personnel Auxiliary to Dentistry. Br J Orthod, 1992; 19: 334-342.
151. Support for the introduction of "professions complimentary to dentistry" was not strong at this time. At the 1997 annual conference of local dental committees held in June 1997 a motion was put "That this conference believes that the Dentist Act must not be amended to expand the role of auxiliaries without the agreement of the profession".
152. Stephens CD, Keith O, Witt P, Sorflett M, Edwards J. Sandy J Orthodontic Auxiliaries - A Pilot Project. Br Dent J 185: 181-187.
153. Health Chiefs bungle delays work. Bristol Evening Post 29th August 1996.
154. Medical academics in funding squeeze. The Guardian June 4th 1996.
155. Clinical Academic Careers – report of an independent tack force (The Richards Report) . Committee of Vice Chancellors and Principals. July 1997
156. Letter to professorial colleagues. July 25th 1996.
157. Mills RW, Uhl A, Blackwell GB, Jandt KD, High power light emitting diode (LED) arrays versus halogen light polymerization of oral biomaterials: Barcol hardness, compressive strength and radiometric properties. Biomaterials 2002; 23: 2955-63.
158. General Dental Council. The first five years: the undergraduate curriculum. General Dental Council, London 1997
159. McDonald DC, Godfrey J. A skills audit for the dental curriculum. European Journal of Dental Education 1999, 3: 167-171.
160. General Dental Council. The First Five Years – A framework for Dental Undergraduate Education General Dental Council , London, 2002.
161. See Obituary. British Dental Journal 1997,182: 442.
162. Leader "Decay of the Dentist. The Times March 25th 1992.
163. The Kings Fund. An independent audit of the NHS under Labour (1997-2005). The Kings Fund .London, April 2005.
164. Long AF, Mercer PE, Stephens CD, Grigg P. The evaluation of three computer assisted learning packages for general dental practitioners. Br Dent J, 1994; 177: 410-415.
165. Grigg P, Stephens CD. A survey of the IT skills and attitudes of final year dental students 1996 and 1997.Europ J Dent Educ 3: 63-74.
166. Grigg P, Macfarlane TV, Shearer AC, Jepson NJA, Stephens CD. Undergraduate computing facilities at 3 UK dental schools in 1997/8, final years students use of them and attitudes to wards information technology. Eur J Dent Educ 2001 5; 101-108.
167. General Dental Council. Recertification and reaccredidation for the dental profession: a consultative document. GDC London, July 1997.
168. Cook J, Stephens CD, .The potential and costs of videoconferencing in dental education in Dental Vocational Training & MFDS Preparation. Annals RCS College and Faculty Bulletin 82: 161-163.
169. Quality Assurance Agency for Higher Education Subject Review Report Q44/2000 University of Bristol: Dentistry http://www.qaa.ac.uk/reviews/reports/subjectLevel/q44_00.pdf
170. Major LE Back on the treadmill . The Guardian 11th January 2000 (http://www.guardian.co.uk/education/2000/jan/11/ highereducation.theguardian?INTCMP=ILCNETTXT3487)
171. Baty P. Millions go down the drain in audit fiasco The Times Higher education Supplement August 4th 2000.
172. Blair A. Speech to the Labour Party Conference September 28th 1999
173. Seward M. Open Wide: Memoir of the Dental Dame. The Memoir Club, Durham, 2009. Page 192.
174. Modernising NHS Dentistry: Implementing the NHS Plan, Department of Health, September 2000.
175. Press Notice, Access to NHS Dentistry. Health Committee. House of Commons, 14th December 2000.
176. Blair T Speech launching Labour's education manifesto at the University of Southampton, 23rd May 2001.
177. Sanders C Selective funding attacked by UUK" Times Higher Education Supplement. Feb 1st 2002.
178. "RAE Rankings come under fire" Times Higher Education Supplement. October 4th 2002.
179. Seward M. Open wide Memoir of the Dental Dame.The Memoir Club Durham, 2009. Chapters 20 and 21.
180. Bedi R Letter NHS Dentistry: Delivering change. Department of Health 19th July 2004.

181. Bartlett E et al. Experiences and perceptions of vocational training reported by the 1999 cohort of vocational dental practitioners on their training in England and Wales. Br Dent J 2001; 191:265-270.
182. Stephens CD, Grigg PA, Greenwod S. Unpublished results.
183. Luther FG.Quality assessment.(Letters) Br Dent J 2004, 196: 4.
184. Clinical academic staffing levels in UK medical and dental schools. The Council of Heads of Medical Schools and the Council of Deans of Dental Schools. May 2004.
185. Modernising Medical Careers. Medically and dentally qualified staff. Recommendations for training the researchers and educators of the future (The Walport Report) .UK Clinical Research Collaboration. March 2005.
186. Cotgreave P. Career Crises (Letter) . Br Dent J 2005, 199: 407.
187. Guys, Kings and St Thomas' incorporating the Royals Dental Hospital!
188. Radford A. The students' year in Newsletter of the Bristol Dental Alumni Association 2007. Page 9.
189. Higher Education Funding Council of England. Development of TQI and the NSS. Letter to Vice Chancellors, 1st November 2006.
190. Rushton VE, Horner K .Academic dentistry. Journal of Dentistry, 2008, 36: 472-480.
191. Stephens CD et al Orthodontic auxiliaries- a pilot project Br Dent J 1998, 185:181-187.
192. See Newsletter of the Bristol Dental Alumni Association 2008,18: 8.
193. Obituary Robert Alexander Darling. British Dental Journal 2011, 210: 47.
194. Grigg J. The Guardian.February 6th. 1969.
195. Saunders CJG. The University of Bristol Dental Hospital and School. Board of Governors of the United Bristol Hospitals, Bristol, 1964. Page 20.
196. Medical Board Minutes. 19th May 1911, Minute 6.
197. Prof Scully acted informally as Head with the agreement of the other clinical professors.
198. Position of Head of School formally agreed by Senate March 1986.